RENAL AND UROLOGIC DISORDERS

VESICOURETERAL REFLUX AND PYELONEPHRITIS

RISK FACTORS, PREVALENCE AND TREATMENT APPROACHES

RENAL AND UROLOGIC DISORDERS

Additional books in this series can be found on Nova's website under the Series tab.

Additional e-books in this series can be found on Nova's website under the e-book tab.

RENAL AND UROLOGIC DISORDERS

VESICOURETERAL REFLUX AND PYELONEPHRITIS

RISK FACTORS, PREVALENCE AND TREATMENT APPROACHES

LEANNA P. NEWPORT
EDITOR

New York

Library of Congress Cataloging-in-Publication Data

ISBN: 978-1-63463-497-7

Library of Congress Control Number: 2014955179

Published by Nova Science Publishers, Inc. † New York

Contents

Preface

Vesicoureteral reflux (VUR) is defined as the retrograde flow of urine from the bladder to the upper urinary tract. It is a common urological entity among children and it is usually diagnosed in the prenatal period or after episodes of febrile urinary tract infection. Reflux can also be found in post-pubertal patients, but it is less common in this population. Pyelonephritis is an upper urinary tract infection involving the kidneys with an incidence in the USA as high as 250.000 cases per year. Most episodes of pyelonephritis are generally considered to be uncomplicated in healthy non pregnant adults. Different risk factors have been identified, such as diabetes, urinary tract obstruction, presence of an indwelling urethral catheter, stent or nephrostomy, functional or anatomic abnormalities of the urinary tract, renal transplantation, immunosuppressive therapy and pregnancy. This book discusses the causes, prevalence and treatment approaches of both VUR and pylonephritis.

Chapter 1 – Pyelonephritis is an upper urinary tract infection involving the kidneys with an incidence in the USA as high as 250.000 cases per year. Most episodes of pyelonephritis are generally considered to be uncomplicated in healthy non pregnant adults. Different risk factors have been identified, such as diabetes, urinary tract obstruction, presence of an indwelling urethral catheter, stent or nephrostomy, functional or anatomic abnormalities of the urinary tract, renal transplantation, immunosuppressive therapy and pregnancy. The microbial spectrum of pyelonephritis consists mainly of ascending urethral infection with Escherichia coli (75 to 95 per cent), and occasional other species of Enterobacteriaceae, such as Proteus mirabilis and Klebsiella pneumonia. In some cases, infection may be due to Staphylococcus aureus or Streptococcus and occur through a haematogenous route. Pseudomonas, Serratia, Providencia species may be responsible for acute complicated pyelonephritis. Clinical manifestations of acute pyelonephritis consist of fever (>38°C), chills, flank pain, and sickness. Patients with acute complicated pyelonephritis may present with sepsis and acute kidney injury. Acute complicated pyelonephritis is the progression of upper urinary tract infection to renal corticomedullary abscess, perinephric abscess, emphysematous pyelonephritis, xanthogranulomatous pyelonephritis, or papillary necrosis. Risk factors for progression to complicated pyelonephritis include anatomic and/or functional abnormalities, urinary tract obstruction, immunosuppression, presence of foreign bodies. Chronic pyelonephritis is commonly due to recurrent infections associated with a chronically obstructing kidney stone (possibly producing xanthogranulomatous pyelonephritis) or vesicoureteral reflux. Affected patients can present with weeks to months of insidious symptoms. Diagnostic evaluation of pyelonephritis requires laboratory workup and radiologic imaging, such as ultrasonograhy, contrast-enhanced ultrasonography, computed tomography and nuclear magnetic resonance. Once diagnosed, pyelonephritis should be treated promptly, initially with empiric antimicrobial therapy, taking into account previous antimicrobial use and results of recent urine cultures, with subsequent adjustment guided by antimicrobial susceptibility data. In this chapter, the author's will review the most important clinical aspects of pyelonephritis, as well as the risk factors and the potential complications of this clinical condition.

Chapter 2 – Vesicoureteral reflux (VUR) is defined as the retrograde flow of urine from the bladder to the upper urinary tract. It is a common urological entity among children and it is usually diagnosed in the prenatal period or after episodes of febrile urinary tract infection. Reflux can also be found in post-pubertal patients, but it is less common in this population. Physicians should be able to recognize and diagnose this pathology, as it is associated with the occurrence of pyelonephritis and renal scarring. In fact, evaluation and treatment of VUR aim at preventing febrile urinary tract infections and renal damage, therefore avoiding further development of reflux nephropathy with hypertension and end-stage renal disease. Different management approaches exist, either surgical or non surgical, and treatment must be tailored to each individual, taking into account patient's characteristics and natural history of VUR. This chapter addresses the aspects regarding the evaluation, diagnosis and management of VUR.

Chapter 3 – Management of vesicoureteral reflux has evolved since the 80's, especially due to the introduction of endoscopic approach. Endoscopic treatment of vesicoureteral reflux has gained popularity because of its minimally invasive character and its favorable success rate. It has become an established alternative to antibiotic prophylaxis and invasive surgical intervention. Literature on subureteral endoscopic injection is growing. Many advances in the indications of treatment, composition of bulking agents and injection techniques have emerged in the past decade. Herein, the author's propose to review indications for endoscopic treatment, technique of injection, different bulking agents and their success rates and finally, adverse events related to their use.

Chapter 4 – *Aim*: Uroplakins (UPs) are urothelium-specific transmembrane proteins consisting of the following four families: uroplakin Ia (UPIa), uroplakin Ib (UPIb), uroplakin II (UPII), and uroplakin III (UPIII). Vesicoureteral reflux (VUR) is the most common congenital urinary tract anomaly. This disease can pose a major threat to the kidneys as twenty percent of patients with endstage renal disease are reported to have VUR. Although genetic studies for *uroplakins* (*UPs*) using mouse have been reported recently, no study has focused on *UP* genes expression in VUR patients. The author's describe here the up-regulation of *UPs* mRNA in exfoliated urinary cells from primary VUR patients. *Methods*: A real-time RT-PCR for *UPs* mRNA was performed on exfoliated urothelial cells from primary VUR and control samples. *UPs* mRNA copies were calculated for each sample. The statistical differences were assessed by the Mann-Whitney U test. Receiver operator characteristic curves were constructed for analysis of the diagnostic values. *Results*: In the tissues, *UPs* gene expressions were significantly up-regulated in VUR samples relative to controls. Considering the author's results, all of the UP gene expressions were up-regulated in the VUR tissues. Moreover, *UPs* mRNA was found to be up-regulated to a greater extent in VUR than in control exfoliated urinary cells. In evaluating the measurement of urinary *UPs* mRNA as a screening test for VUR, the sensitivity and the specificity could be determined by the best diagnostic cutoff point. *Discussion*: Regarding *UPs* mRNA in VUR, two studies of *UPII* and *UPIII* gene knockout mouse models were reported. All of the unaffected *UP* transcripts were shown by Northern blotting to be up-regulated. Though these studies were in mice, the findings are compatible with the author's results in humans. The author's studies may have less impact because the control subjects were not age-matched. However, the author's submit that UPs and the author's results can lead to clarifying the etiology of VUR in the future. Further studies are needed of samples obtained from age- adjusted pediatric patients with other urological conditions, such as cystitis, pyelonephritis, and congenital hydronephrosis. The author's also investigated by a (99m) technetium dimercaptosuccinic acid renal scan the relationship between *UP* mRNA expression and the degree of renal scarring in

VUR tissue samples. Although not significant, higher expression levels were found for *UP* mRNAs with the increasing degree of renal scarring. These results show the feasibility of quantitative measurements for urinary *UP* mRNAs and the potential use in screening for VUR. In addition, the author's preliminary studies of RT-PCR for tissue *UP* mRNAs can be useful in elucidating the underlying mechanisms leading to VUR in the future. *Conclusions*: The author's submit that the quantitative measurement of urinary *Ups* mRNA has a potential of developing into the first non-invasive screening test for VUR.

In: Vesicoureteral Reflux and Pyelonephritis ISBN: 978-1-63463-497-7
Editor: Leanna P. Newport

Chapter I

Pyelonephritis: Epidemiology, Pathogenesis and Management

***Anna Clementi, M.D.*[1,*], *Viviana Rosalia Scarfia, M.D.*[1], *Monica Insalaco, M.D.*[1], *Pasquale Fatuzzo, M.D.*[2] and *Antonio Granata, M.D.*[1]**

[1]Nephrology and Dialysis Unit, "San Giovanni di Dio" Hospital, Agrigento, Italy

[2]Nephrology and Dialysis Unit, University Hospital of Catania, Italy

Abstract

Pyelonephritis is an upper urinary tract infection involving the kidneys with an incidence in the USA as high as 250.000 cases per year. Most episodes of pyelonephritis are generally considered to be uncomplicated in healthy non pregnant adults. Different risk factors have been identified, such as diabetes, urinary tract obstruction, presence of an indwelling urethral catheter, stent or nephrostomy, functional or anatomic abnormalities of the urinary tract, renal transplantation, immunosuppressive therapy and pregnancy. The microbial spectrum of pyelonephritis consists mainly of ascending urethral infection with

[*] *Anna Clementi:* a.clementi81@virgilio.it,

Escherichia coli (75 to 95 per cent), and occasional other species of Enterobacteriaceae, such as Proteus mirabilis and Klebsiella pneumonia. In some cases, infection may be due to Staphylococcus aureus or Streptococcus and occur through a haematogenous route. Pseudomonas, Serratia, Providencia species may be responsible for acute complicated pyelonephritis. Clinical manifestations of acute pyelonephritis consist of fever (>38°C), chills, flank pain, and sickness. Patients with acute complicated pyelonephritis may present with sepsis and acute kidney injury. Acute complicated pyelonephritis is the progression of upper urinary tract infection to renal corticomedullary abscess, perinephric abscess, emphysematous pyelonephritis, xanthogranulomatous pyelonephritis, or papillary necrosis. Risk factors for progression to complicated pyelonephritis include anatomic and/or functional abnormalities, urinary tract obstruction, immunosuppression, presence of foreign bodies. Chronic pyelonephritis is commonly due to recurrent infections associated with a chronically obstructing kidney stone (possibly producing xanthogranulomatous pyelonephritis) or vesicoureteral reflux. Affected patients can present with weeks to months of insidious symptoms. Diagnostic evaluation of pyelonephritis requires laboratory workup and radiologic imaging, such as ultrasonograhy, contrast-enhanced ultrasonography, computed tomography and nuclear magnetic resonance. Once diagnosed, pyelonephritis should be treated promptly, initially with empiric antimicrobial therapy, taking into account previous antimicrobial use and results of recent urine cultures, with subsequent adjustment guided by antimicrobial susceptibility data. In this chapter, we will review the most important clinical aspects of pyelonephritis, as well as the risk factors and the potential complications of this clinical condition.

Epidemiology

Acute pyelonephritis (APN) is an infection of the upper urinary tract, specifically the renal parenchyma and renal pelvis. APN is considered uncomplicated if the infection is caused by a typical pathogen in a immunocompetent patient who has normal urinary tract anatomy and renal function. APN in the USA has an incidence as high as 250,000 cases per year and requires 100,000 hospitalizations every year [1]. Approximately 20% to 35% of females experience an episode of APN in their lifetime [2]. Even though women are five times more likely than men to be hospitalized with this condition (11.7 versus 2.4 hospitalizations per 10,000 cases, respectively), they seem to have a lower mortality rate than males (7.3 versus 16.5 deaths per

1,000 cases, respectively) [3]. Acute pyelonephritis occurs in 1 to 2 percent of pregnant women, increasing the risk for premature labor and low-birth-weight infants [4]. Moreover, APN is one of the most common causes of post-transplantation urinary tract infection with a high incidence of morbidity and graft failure. Valera et al. reported 21 episodes per 100 patients-years of acute pyelonephritis among 161 kidney recipients [5]. In the study of Pellé et al., 18.7% of the renal transplant recipients with urinary tract infections went on to develop APN, which was calculated to be an independent risk factor for deterioration of renal graft function [6].

Risk Factors and Pathogenesis

Different risk factors for acute pyelonephritis have been identified, such as female gender, diabetes mellitus, postmenopausal state, previous recurrent urinary tract infections, urinary tract obstruction, presence of an indwelling urethral catheter, stent or nephrostomy, functional or anatomic abnormalities of the urinary tract (vesicoureteral reflux, in particular), renal transplantation, immunosuppressive therapy and pregnancy [7]. Moreover, a genetic predisposition to APN has been suggested by the strong association between a history of urinary tract infection in one or more first-degree female relatives and an increased risk of recurrent cystitis and pyelonephritis [8]. Marked familial clustering of cases of APN among the relatives of pyelonephritis-prone children, associated with significantly lower expression of CXCR1, an interleukin-8 receptor [9]. In kidney transplanted patients, female gender, acute rejection episodes and the number of recurrent urinary tract infections seem to represent independent risk factors associated with APN [6].

Most renal parenchymal infections occur secondary to bacterial ascent through the urethra and urinary bladder. Haematogenous acute pyelonephritis occurs most often in debilitated, chronically ill patients and those receiving immunosuppressive therapy.

In more than 80 percent of cases of acute pyelonephritis, the etiologic agent is Escherichia coli [10]. Uropathogenic Escherichia coli are a specific subset of extraintestinal pathogenic Escherichia coli, whose virulence factors include fimbriae, flagella, diverse adhesions, siderophores and toxins able to subvert host defenses and stimulate an inflammatory response [11,12]. In elderly patients, Escherichia coli is a less common (60 percent) cause of acute pyelonephritis. The increased use of catheters and instruments among these patients predisposes them to infections with other gram-negative organisms such as Proteus, Klebsiella, Serratia, or Pseudomonas [1]. In diabetic patients Klebsiella, Enterobacter, Clostridium and Candida are the most common causes of acute pyelonephritis, which might complicate and lead to renal failure [13,14]. Haematogenous infection is invariably due to Staphylococcus aureus or Streptococcus species [15].

Table 1. Risk factors for acute complicated pyelonephritis

AGE Infants Elderly (>60 years)	**IMMUNOSUPPRESSED STATE** Diabetes Transplantation Malignancy Sickle cell disease Chemoradiation HIV infection Corticosteroid use
ANATOMIC/FUNCTIONAL ABNORMALITIES Policystic Kidney Disease Horeshoe Kidney Double Ureter Ureterocele Vescicoureteric reflux	**OBSTRUCTION** Calculi Bladder neck obstruction Posterior urethral valve Benign prostatic hypertrophy Neurogenic bladder
FOREIGN BODY Indwelling urethral catheter Stent Nephrostomy tube Urinary diversion	**PREGNANCY**

Acute complicated pyelonephritis is the progression of upper urinary tract infection to renal corticomedullary abscess, perinephric abscess, emphysematous pyelonephritis, xanthogranulomatous pyelonephritis, or papillary necrosis. Risk factors for complicated acute pyelonephritis are those that increase susceptibility or reduce host response to infections (Table 1) [13,16].

Renal abscess can develop both in case of haematogenous spread and in the setting of ascending infection from the bladder [17]. Diabetes mellitus, anatomical abnormalities in the urinary tract, such as vesicoureteral reflux, and renal stones are known risk factors for its development. Perinephric abscess may be a consequence of the disruption of a corticomedullary renal abscess or an obstructing renal pelvic stone.[17,18]. Kidney emphysematous complications are likely to be due to the presence of organisms which rapidly ferment glucose and produce carbon dioxide. Impaired transport of metabolic end products due to impaired tissue perfusion in case of diabetes contribute as well [19]. Immunosuppression and diabetes may also predispose to the development of xanthogranulomatous pyelonephritis, where the destroyed renal tissue is replaced by hard, yellow xanthogranulomatous material. Chronic renal obstruction and infection, alterations in lipid metabolism, lymphatic obstruction, and renal ischemia may play an important role in the pathogenesis of this clinical condition [20,21].

Finally, papillary necrosis seems to be due to a marginal change in vascular supply leading to infarction and sloughing of papillae. Risk factors for its development include diabetes, sickle cell disease and obstructive uropathy [22].

Clinical Presentation and Outcomes

The spectrum of acute pyelonephritis is wide, ranging from a mild illness to sepsis syndrome [13]. Clinical manifestations suggestive of APN include fever (temperature >38°C), chills, flank pain, costovertebral-angle tenderness, and nausea or vomiting. Symptoms that are suggestive of cystitis, such as dysuria, urinary bladder frequency and urgency, suprapubic pain and haematuria, may be also present. In some cases, the presentation may mimic pelvic inflammatory disease. In the study of Pinson et al. performed on young and middle-aged women presenting to an emergency department with fever, pyuria, and other features of upper urinary tract infection, 98 percent had acute pyelonephritis [23]. In the absence of fever, 16 percent were given alternative diagnoses.

However, in 20% of elderly patients acute pyelonephritis may present with gastrointestinal or pulmonary symptoms and up to one third of them have no fever [13]. Moreover, fever and leukocytosis are of little value in diagnosing acute pyelonephritis in patients who have indwelling bladder catheters, especially when infections are caused by gram-positive cocci or Candida [24]. The differential diagnosis of acute pyelonephritis includes pelvic inflammatory disease, cholecystitis, appendicitis, lower lobe pneumonia, perforated viscus, and the prodrome of herpes zoster [1].

Up to 30 percent of women presenting with cystitis-like symptoms have upper urinary tract involvement (subclinical pyelonephritis), but these infections rarely cause any cortical damage. Pregnancy, recurrent urinary tract infections, diabetes and immunosuppression may predispose to this clinical condition [16].

Renal transplant recipients with urinary tract infections are more likely to be clinically asymptomatic compared to non-immunocompromised patients, and do not mount the typical inflammatory response to infection as a consequence of immunosuppression [25].

On the other hand, urinary tract infections are often associated with acute pyelonephritis and rapidly developing bacteraemia potentially progressing to the full-blown picture of urosepsis, particularly during the early post-transplant period [25]. Even though APN is not associated with an increased risk of mortality in transplanted patients, it seems to impair long term allograft function [6]. Giral et al. found that early, but not late, recurrent APN was significantly associated with graft loss possibly by inducing or accelerating graft fibrosis [26].

Patients with acute complicated pyelonephritis may present with sepsis, multiple organ system dysfunction, shock, and acute renal failure [27]. In some cases, complicated pyelonephritis may be associated with weeks to months of insidious, nonspecific signs and symptoms such as malaise, fatigue, nausea, or abdominal pain [27]. Chronic pyelonephritis is commonly due to recurrent infections associated with a chronically obstructing kidney stone (possibly producing xanthogranulomatous pyelonephritis) or vesicoureteral reflux. Affected patients can present with anorexia, fatigue and weight loss.

Diagnosis

Acute pyelonephritis should be suspected in case of fever, chills, flank pain, costovertebral-angle tenderness, and nausea or vomiting, supported by laboratory evidence of pyuria and/or bacteriuria. Assessment for pyuria and bacteriuria is often performed with the use of commercially available dipsticks that test for leukocyte esterase and for nitrites [28]. The dipstick test is most accurate for predicting urinary tract infection when the presence of either leukocyte esterase or nitrite is considered a positive result, with a sensitivity of 75% and a specificity of 82% [29,30]. However, results of the dipstick test provide little useful information when the history is strongly suggestive of urinary tract infection, since even negative results for both tests do not reliably rule out the infection in such cases [29]. Haematuria may be also present [31].

A urine culture is performed to confirm the presence of bacteriuria and the antimicrobial susceptibility of the infecting uropathogen [28]. It is positive in 90 percent of patients with acute pyelonephritis, and it should be obtained before initiation of antibiotic therapy [1].

Even though, 20% of hospitalized patients have positive blood cultures [13], there is no evidence that they indicate a more complicated course in otherwise healthy persons with APN [32]. Therefore, blood cultures are indicated only if there is diagnostic uncertainty, the patient is immune-suppressed, or a haematogenous source is suspected [33,34].

Imaging is not routinely indicated in patients with acute pyelonephritis and treatment can be started based on typical clinical and laboratory features [35]. A radiological evaluation is required early for patients with severe symptoms, high-risk cases (including the elderly, diabetics, immune-compromised patients and transplant recipients) and those who do not respond to i.v. antibiotic therapy within 72 hours [36].

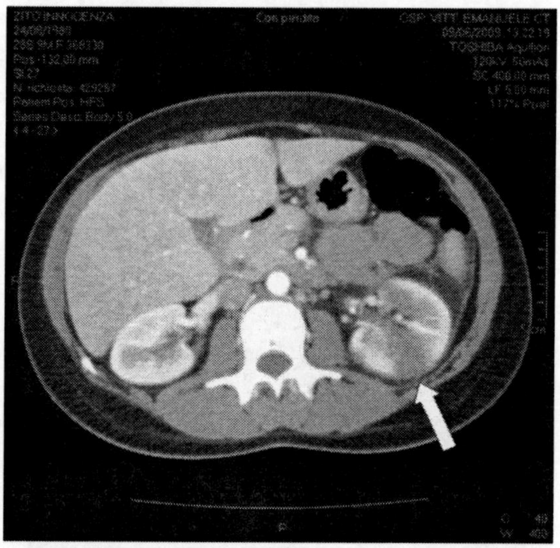

Figure 1. Contrast-enhanced CT scan showing soft hypoenhanced area in the renal parenchyma of the left kidney (white arrow).

Contrast-enhanced computed tomography (CT) is considered the imaging method of choice in the diagnosis of APN [37]. Unenhanced CT can detect calculi, gas formation, haemorrhage, parenchymal calcifications, obstruction, renal enlargement and inflammatory masses [35,38] and therefore should be performed initially, although the kidney often appears normal [38,39]. The most common radiologic contrast-enhanced CT finding of APN is a striated or wedge-shaped area of hypoperfusion or mass-like lesion after contrast injection (Figure 1) [40,41]. This area of hypoperfusion is formed by obstruction of blood vessels resulting from spasm, edema of the interstitium, and the presence of intraluminal inflammatory metabolites [42]. Acute pyelonephritis areas may have a lobar distribution and may be unifocal, multifocal or bilateral.

Other CT signs of pyelonephritis include focal or global enlargement of the kidney, obliteration of the renal sinus and perinephric fat planes, stranding, thickening of Gerota's fascia, and calyceal effacement caused by swelling of adjacent parenchyma and thickening of the pelvicalyceal wall [35,38,43]. Other uncommon radiologic findings such as perirenal fat infiltration, ureteral wall edema, renal abscess formation, pelvic ascites, portal edema, and renal scarring are also observed on CT scans [42, 44].

In case of emphysematous pyelonephritis, CT is able to detect gas and to define the extent of the disease. Parenchymal gas typically appears as multiple small bubbles or linear streaks radiating from the papillae as the gas dissects along planes of the interstitium [39]. Other CT findings include larger locules of gas, perirenal fluid, gas–fluid levels, abscesses and parenchymal destruction [15]. In the setting of xanthogranulomatous pyelonephritis, typical CT features include enlarged, non-functioning kidneys, containing multiple rounded, hypoattenuating masses typically arranged in a hydronephrotic pattern [38].

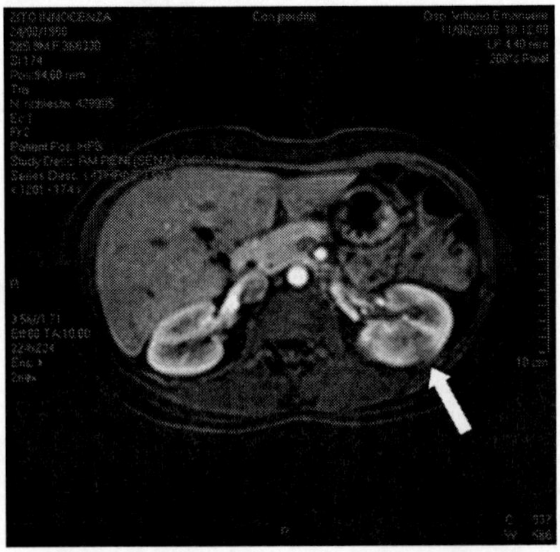

Figure 2. s4THRIVE DYN MRI scan (T1-w) showing a focal area of APN (white arrow).

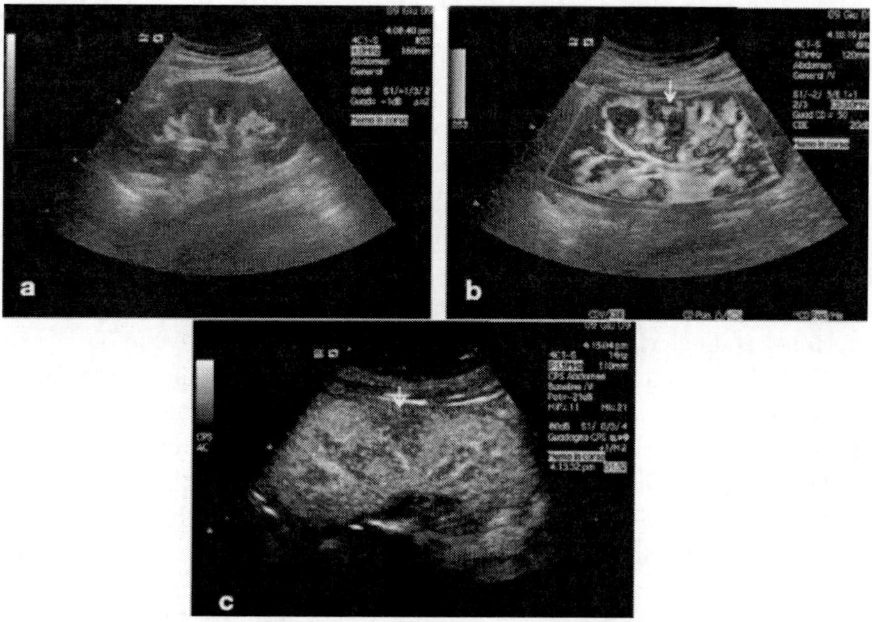

Figure 3. a) B-mode ultrasonography does not show any structural kidney abnormalities. b) Power-Doppler use reveals a hypoperfused area of APN (white arrow). c) Longitudinal scan: Contrast-Enhanced Ultrasound showing 15s after contrast injection a clear wedge-shaped area (white arrow) of hypoperfusion due to acute pyelonephritis in the mesorenal region.

Even though contrast-enhanced CT scanning is advocated as the most rewarding investigation of acute pyelonephritis, it exposes the patient to radiation and requires iodinated contrast medium administration with its possible side effects on renal function [45].

Renal cortical scintigraphy, using 99mTc-DMSA, offers relatively high-resolution images of the cortex and it is the imaging method of choice in paediatric patients [46].

The absence of ionizing radiation or iodinated contrast agents, coupled with technological advances, have contributed to the increasing acceptance of magnetic resonance imaging (MRI) as an alternative to CT in the study of acute pyelonephritis, especially in pregnant women or women of childbearing age and patients with contraindications to iodinated contrast agents [47,48]. As with CT, dynamic MRI with gadolinium chelates allows for morphological and functional evaluation of inflammatory renal disease and its potential complications [49]. Common MRI findings in the setting of APN include increased renal volume, focal or diffuse signal alterations on baseline scans, areas of non-enhancement after contrast administration, presence of abscess foci, extrarenal spread of the inflammatory process and urinary tract dilatation (Figure 2) [50].

There are, however, potential pitfalls related to MRI. Gas-forming infections and calculi can cause signal voids which are difficult to interpret. While these are rare in children [51], they are common in adults and can limit the value of MRI. Moreover, MRI with gadolinium chelates may predispose patients with a glomerular filtration rate ≤ 30 ml/min to the development of nephrogenic cutaneous fibrosis. In patients with reduced kidney function, diffusion-weighted MRI can be considered as a valid alternative [47].

Conventional ultrasonography (US) has only limited value, especially in the absence of calicopyelic ectasy, in the diagnosis of acute pyelonephritis, with a very low sensitivity (11-40%) for detecting renal parenchymal lesions [37] (Figure 3a). It is mainly used to exclude urinary complications, such as tract obstruction or abscess [52]. Doppler US improves the sensitivity for detecting the parenchymal changes in the setting of APN from 38% to 63% [53]. Power Doppler US has higher sensitivity and specificity compared to colour Doppler US, especially in children (Figure 3b) [36, 54, 55]. However, power Doppler US presents some limitations in the detection of low flow and might miss renal parenchymal changes in APN [56]. The advent of newer US contrast agents has improved the detection of hypoperfused renal areas in the setting of acute pyelonephritis. Contrast-enhanced US (CEUS) is able, indeed, to improve the detection of low flow by improving the signal-to-noise ratio (Figure 3c) [57]. CEUS presents several advantages in patients with chronic kidney disease, such as low cost and low toxicity, combined with a good diagnostic performance in terms of sensibility, specificity, accuracy and positive predictive value [58].

In spite of technical ultrasonographic improvements, contrast-enhanced tomography remains the reference standard for both the diagnosis and follow-up of acute pyelonephritis [37].

Management

Most episodes of acute uncomplicated pyelonephritis are now treated in the outpatient setting [59,60]. A urine culture should be performed before the initiation of antibiotic therapy to guide treatment. Of the common uropathogens, resistance to fluoroquinolones remains very low (1 to 3 percent) [61].

Therefore, for empiric therapy in uncomplicated acute pyelonephritis, the Infectious Disease Society of America (IDSA) recommends the use of an oral fluoroquinolone (Table 2) [62], which should be avoided in pregnant women. Oral amoxicillin-clavulanate and trimethoprim-sulfamethoxazole provide acceptable alternatives for susceptible organisms (Table 2) [62].

Table 2. Outpatient empirical treatment of acute uncomplicated pyelonephritis. ISDA=Infectious Disease Society of America

FLUOROQUINOLONES
•Ciprofloxacin 500 mg given orally twice daily or 1 gr given orally once daily for 7 days
•Levofloxacin 750 mg given orally once daily for 5 days
TRIMETHOPRIM-SULFAMETHOXAZOLE
160 and 800 mg orally twice daily for 14 days
ORAL BETA-LACTAMS
Specific agents not listed in IDSA guidelines for 10 to 14 days

Patients with complicated acute pyelonephritis who are more ill or have not responded to outpatient therapy should be hospitalized. The IDSA guidelines recommend one of three initial intravenous therapies: (1) a fluoroquinolone; (2) an aminoglycoside with or without ampicillin; or (3) an extended-spectrum cephalosporin with or without an aminoglycoside [62]. Anyway, aminoglycosides are contraindicated in case of pre-existing renal disease. Oral treatment is feasible as soon as the patient becomes afebrile, has improved clinically, and can tolerate oral hydration and medications [1]. A seven- to 14-day course of antibiotics is effective in immunocompetent patients [13,61], while APN in the setting of immunosuppressive states responds well to a 14- to 21-day course of a fluoroquinolone or TMP-SMX [16]. Post-treatment urine cultures are recommended in all patients at the follow-up visit, one to two weeks after completion of antibiotic therapy [63].

The two most common causes of initial treatment failure are resistant organisms and nephrolithiasis. Imaging studies may be useful in case of complicated acute pyelonephritis. Immediate release of any existing obstruction combined with a 14-day course of appropriate antibiotics minimizes failure and recurrence of the infection [16]. Relief of obstruction and antibiotic therapy may be successful in emphysematous pyelonephritis, but nephrectomy must be strongly considered in patients with unresponsive infections [13].

If parenchymal involvement including abscesses is observed, longer courses of antibiotics (intravenous or oral) or sequential therapy may be necessary. Pregnant women and transplanted patients with pyelonephritis require hospitalization (for at least a short observation period) for aggressive hydration and parenteral antibiotics. Antibiotic treatment is similar to the treatments of other adult regimens [1].

Conclusion

Acute pyelonephritis is a relative frequent clinical condition in women and in immunosuppressed patients. Its diagnosis remains predominantly clinical, supported by imaging studies in complicated cases. Therapy should initiated promptly to avoid both worsening of clinical conditions and the development of severe complications.

References

[1] Ramakrishnan K, Scheid DC. Diagnosis and management of acute pyelonephritis in adults. *Am. Fam. Physician.,* 2005 Mar 1;71(5):933-42.

[2] Jung YH, Cho IR, Lee SE, Lee KC, Kim JG, Jeon JS, et al. Comparative analysis of clinical parameters in acute pyelonephritis. *Korean J. Urol.,* 2007;48:29-34.

[3] Foxman B, Klemstine KL, Brown PD. Acute pyelonephritis in US hospitals in 1997: hospitalization and in-hospital mortality. *Ann. Epidemiol.,* 2003;13:144-50.

[4] Gilstrap LC 3d, Ramin SM. Urinary tract infections during pregnancy. *Obstet. Gynecol. Clin. North Am.,* 2001;28:581-91.

[5] Valera B, Gentil MA, Cabello V, Fijo J, Cordero E, Cisneros JM. Epidemiology of urinary infections in renal transplant recipients. *Transplant Proc.,* 2006 Oct;38(8):2414-5.

[6] Pellé G, Vimont S, Levy PP, Hertig A, Ouali N, Chassin C, Arlet G, Rondeau E, Vandewalle A. Acute pyelonephritis represents a risk factor impairing long-term kidney graft function. *Am. J. Transplant.,* 2007 Apr; 7(4):899-907.

[7] Scholes D, Hooton TM, Roberts PL, Gupta K, Stapleton AE, Stamm WE. Risk factors associated with acute pyelonephritis in healthy women. *Ann. Intern. Med.,* 2005;142:20-7.

[8] Scholes D, Hawn TR, Roberts PL, Li SS, Stapleton AE, Zhao LP, Stamm WE, Hooton TM. Family history and risk of recurrent cystitis and pyelonephritis in women. *J. Urol.,* 2010 Aug;184(2):564-9.

[9] Lundstedt AC, Leijonhufvud I, Ragnarsdottir B, Karpman D, Andersson B, Svanborg C. Inherited susceptibility to acute pyelonephritis: a family study of urinary tract infection. *J. Infect. Dis.,* 2007 Apr 15;195(8):1227-34.

[10] Stamm WE, Hooton TM. Management of urinary tract infections in adults. *N. Engl. J. Med.,* 1993;329:1328-34.

[11] Johnson JR. Microbial virulence determinants and the pathogenesis of urinarytract infection. *Infect. Dis. Clin. North Am.,* 2003 Jun;17(2):261-78.

[12] Nielubowicz GR, Mobley HL. Host-pathogen interactions in urinary tract infection. *Nat. Rev. Urol.,* 2010 Aug;7(8):430-41.

[13] Bass PF 3d, Jarvis JA, Mitchell CK. Urinary tract infections. *Prim. Care,* 2003;30:41-61.

[14] Roberts JA. Management of pyelonephritis and upper urinary tract infections. *Urol. Clin. North Am.,* 1999;26:753-63.

[15] Papanicolaou N, Pfister RC. Acute renal infections. *Radiol. Clin. North Am.,* 1996;34:965–995.

[16] Bergeron MG. Treatment of pyelonephritis in adults. *Med. Clin. North Am.,* 1995;79:619-49.

[17] Fowler JE, Jr, Perkins T. Presentation, diagnosis and treatment of renal abscesses: 1972-1988. *J. Urol.,* 1994;151:847–51.

[18] Coelho RF, Schneider-Monteiro ED, Mesquita JL, Mazzucchi E, Marmo Lucon A, Srougi M. Renal and perinephric abscesses: Analysis of 65 consecutive cases. *World J. Surg.,* 2007;31:431–6.

[19] Huang JJ, Tseng CC. Emphesematous pyelonephritis: Clinico-radiological classification, management, prognosis, and pathogenesis. *Arch. Intern. Med.,* 2000;160:797–805.

[20] Li L, Parwani AV. Xanthogranulomatous pyelonephritis. *Arch. Pathol. Lab. Med.,* 2011;135:671–4.

[21] Loffroy R, Guiu B, Watfa J, Michel F, Cercueil JP, Krausé D. Xanthogranulomatous pyelonephritis in adults: Clinical and radiological findings in diffuse and focal forms. *Clin. Radiol.,* 2007;62:884–90.

[22] Griffin MD, Bergstalhn EJ, Larson TS. Renal papillary necrosis: A sixteen year clinical experience. *J. Am. Soc. Nephrol.,* 1995;6:248–56.

[23] Pinson AG, Philbrick JT, Lindbeck GH, Schorling JB. Fever in the clinical diagnosis of acute pyelonephritis. *Am. J. Emerg. Med.,* 1997;15: 148-51.

[24] Tambyah PA, Maki DG. Catheter-associated urinary tract infection is rarely symptomatic: a prospective study of 1,497 catheterized patients. *Arch. Intern. Med.,* 2000;160:678-82.

[25] Säemann M, Hörl WH. Urinary tract infection in renal transplant recipients. *Eur. J. Clin. Invest.,* 2008 Oct;38 Suppl 2:58-65.

[26] Giral M, Pascuariello G, Karam G, Hourmant M, Cantarovich D, Dantal J, Blancho G, Coupel S, Josien R, Daguin P, Méchineau S, Soulillou JP. Acute graft pyelonephritis and long-term kidney allograft outcome. *Kidney Int.,* 2002 May;61(5):1880-6.

[27] Mnif MF, Kamoun M, Kacem FH, Bouaziz Z, Charfi N, Mnif F, Naceur BB, Rekik N, Abid M. Complicated urinary tract infections associated with diabetes mellitus: Pathogenesis, diagnosis and management. *Indian J. Endocrinol. Metab.,* 2013 May;17(3):442-5.

[28] Hooton TM. Clinical practice. Uncomplicated urinary tract infection. *N. Engl. J. Med.,* 2012 Mar 15;366(11):1028-37.

[29] Bent S, Nallamothu BK, Simel DL, Fihn SD, Saint S. Does this woman have an acute uncomplicated urinary tract infection? *JAMA,* 2002 May 22-29;287(20):2701-10.

[30] Hurlbut TA 3rd, Littenberg B. The diagnostic accuracy of rapid dipstick tests to predict urinary tract infection. *Am. J. Clin. Pathol.,* 1991 Nov;96 (5): 582-8.

[31] Hooton TM, Stamm WE. Diagnosis and treatment of uncomplicated urinary tract infection. Infect Dis Clin North Am 1997;11:551-81.

[32] Miller O 2d, Hemphill RR. Urinary tract infection and pyelonephritis. *Emerg. Med. Clin. North Am.,* 2001;19: 655-74.

[33] McMurray BR, Wrenn KD, Wright SW. Usefulness of blood cultures in pyelonephritis. *Am. J. Emerg. Med.,* 1997;15:137-40.

[34] Velasco M, Martinez JA, Moreno-Martinez A, Horcajada JP, Ruiz J, Barranco M, et al. Blood cultures for women with uncomplicated acute pyelonephritis: are they necessary? *Clin. Infect. Dis.,* 2003;37:1127-30.

[35] Kawashima A, Sandler CM, Goldman SM. Imaging in acute renal infection. *BJU Int.,* 2000 Jul;86 Suppl 1:70-9.

[36] Browne RF, Zwirewich C, Torreggiani WC. Imaging of urinary tract infection in the adult. *Eur. Radiol.,* 2004 Mar;14 Suppl 3:E168-83.

[37] Mitterberger M, Pinggera GM, Colleselli D, Bartsch G, Strasser H, Steppan I, Pallwein L, Friedrich A, Gradl J, Frauscher F. Acute pyelonephritis: comparison of diagnosis with computed tomography and contrast-enhanced ultrasonography. *BJU Int.,* 2008 Feb;101(3):341-4.

[38] Kawashima A, Sandler CM, Ernst RD, Goldman SM, Raval B, Fishman EK (1997) Renal inflammatory disease: the current role of CT. *Crit. Rev. Diagn Imaging,* 38:369–415.

[39] Kaplan DM, Rosenfield AT, Smith RC (1997) Advances in the imaging of renal infection. Helical CT and modern coordinated imaging. *Infect. Dis. Clin. North Am.,* 11:681–705.

[40] Soulen MC, Fishman EK, Goldman SM, Gatewood OM. Bacterial renal infection: role of CT. *Radiology,* 1989;171:703-7.

[41] Gold RP, McClennan BL, Rottenberg RR. CT appearance of acute inflammatory disease of the renal interstitium. *AJR Am. J. Roentgenol.,* 1983;141:343-9.

[42] Talner LB, Davidson AJ, Lebowitz RL, Dalla Palma L, Goldman SM. Acute pyelonephritis: can we agree on terminology? *Radiology,* 1994; 192:297-305.

[43] Baumgarten DA, Baumgartner BR (1997) Imaging and radiologic management of upper urinary tract infections.Urol Clin North Am 24:545–569

[44] Tsugaya M, Hirao N, Sakagami H, Ohtaguro K, Washida H. Renal cortical scarring in acute pyelonephritis. *Br. J. Urol.,* 1992;69:245-9.

[45] Kraus SJ (2001) Genitourinary imaging in children. *Pediatr. Clin. North Am.,* 48:1381–1424.

[46] Granata A, Floccari F, Insalaco M, Clementi A, Di Lullo L, D'Amelio A, Zamboli P, Logias F, Romano M, Fiorini F. L'ecografia nelle infezioni del rene. *GIN,* 2012;29(S57): S47-S57.

[47] Stunell H, Buckley O, Feeney J, Geoghegan T, Browne RF, Torreggiani WC. Imaging of acute pyelonephritis in the adult. *Eur. Radiol.,* 2007 Jul;17(7):1820-8.

[48] Rusinek H, Kaur M, Lee VS. Renal magnetic resonance imaging. *Curr. Opin. Nephrol. Hypertens,* 2004 Nov;13(6):667-73.

[49] Israel GM. MRI of the kidney and urinary tract. *J. Magn. Reson Imaging,* 2006 Oct;24(4):725-34.

[50] Martina MC, Campanino PP, Caraffo F, Marcuccio C, Gunetti F, Colla L, Cassinis MC, Gandini G. Dynamic magnetic resonance imaging in acute pyelonephritis. *Radiol. Med.,* 2010 Mar;115(2):287-300.

[51] Majd M, Nussbaum-Blask AR,Markle BM et al. (2001) Acute pyelonephritis: comparison of diagnosis with 99m Tc-DMSA SPECT, spiral CT,MR imaging, and power-Doppler US in an experimental pig model. *Radiology,* 218:101–108.

[52] Noble VE, Brown DF. Renal ultrasound. *Emerg. Med. Clin. North Am.,* 2004;22:641-59.

[53] Eggli KD, Eggli D. Color Doppler sonography in pyelonephritis. *Pediatr. Radiol.,* 1992;22(6):422-5.

[54] Basiratnia M, Noohi AH, Lotfi M, Alavi MS. Power Doppler sonographic evaluation of acute childhood pyelonephritis. *Pediatr. Nephrol.,* 2006 Dec;21(12):1854-7.

[55] Halevy R, Smolkin V, Bykov S, Chervinsky L, Sakran W, Koren A. Power Doppler ultrasonography in the diagnosis of acute childhood pyelonephritis. *Pediatr. Nephrol.,* 2004 Sep;19(9):987-91.

[56] Clautice-Engle T, Jeffrey RB Jr. Renal hypoperfusion: value of power Doppler imaging. *AJR Am. J. Roentgenol.,* 1997 May;168(5):1227-31.

[57] Correas JM, Claudon M, Tranquart F, Hélénon AO. The kidney: imaging with microbubble contrast agents. Ultrasound Q. 2006 Mar; 22(1):53-66.

[58] Granata A, Andrulli S, Fiorini F, Basile A, Logias F, Figuera M, Sicurezza E, Gallieni M, Fiore CE. Diagnosis of acute pyelonephritis by contrast-enhanced ultrasonography in kidney transplant patients. *Nephrol. Dial Transplant.,* 2011 Feb;26(2):715-20.

[59] Czaja CA, Scholes D, Hooton TM, Stamm WE. Population-based epidemiologic analysis of acute pyelonephritis. *Clin. Infect. Dis.,* 2007 Aug 1;45(3):273-80.

[60] Nicolle LE. Uncomplicated urinary tract infection in adults including uncomplicated pyelonephritis. *Urol. Clin. North Am.,* 2008 Feb;35(1):1-12.

[61] Nicolle LE. Urinary tract infection: traditional pharmacologic therapies. *Am. J. Med.,* 2002;113(suppl 1A): 35S-44S.

[62] Warren JW, Abrutyn E, Hebel JR, Johnson JR, Schaeffer AJ, Stamm WE. Guidelines for antimicrobial treatment of uncomplicated acute bacterial cystitis and acute pyelonephritis in women. Infectious Diseases Society of America (IDSA). *Clin. Infect. Dis.,* 1999;29:745-58.

[63] Delzell JE JR, Fitzsimmons A. Urinary tract infection. The American Board of Family Practice. Reference Guide. 7th ed. American Board of Family Practice, 2001. Accessed online December 5, 2004, at: http://www.abfp.org/guides/UTI.pdf

In: Vesicoureteral Reflux and Pyelonephritis ISBN: 978-1-63463-497-7
Editor: Leanna P. Newport

Chapter II

Vesicoureteral Reflux: Diagnosis and Treatment

Michelle Bergeron, Anne-Sophie Blais, Stéphane Bolduc and Katherine Moore*
Division of Urology, Department of Surgery,
CHU de Québec Université Laval, Québec, Canada

Abstract

Vesicoureteral reflux (VUR) is defined as the retrograde flow of urine from the bladder to the upper urinary tract. It is a common urological entity among children and it is usually diagnosed in the prenatal period or after episodes of febrile urinary tract infection. Reflux can also be found in post-pubertal patients, but it is less common in this population. Physicians should be able to recognize and diagnose this pathology, as it is associated with the occurrence of pyelonephritis and renal scarring. In fact, evaluation and treatment of VUR aim at preventing febrile urinary tract infections and renal damage, therefore avoiding further development of reflux nephropathy with hypertension and end-stage renal disease. Different management approaches exist, either surgical or non surgical, and treatment must be tailored to each

* Corresponding author: Katherine Moore, MD, FRCSC, CHU de Québec, Pavillon CHUL 2705 Boul Laurier R-1742, Québec, Québec, Canada, G1V 4G2, Tel: 418-654-2282, Fax: 418-654-2137, katherine.moore.1@ulaval.ca.

individual, taking into account patient's characteristics and natural history of VUR. This chapter addresses the aspects regarding the evaluation, diagnosis and management of VUR.

Introduction

Vesicoureteral reflux (VUR) is defined as the retrograde flow of urine from the bladder into the upper urinary tract. VUR is a common urological finding among children and is usually diagnosed in the prenatal period or after episodes of febrile urinary tract infection (UTI). The clinical importance of VUR lies in its association with an increased risk of recurrent pyelonephritis and renal scarring, which can ultimately result in early hypertension and end stage renal disease. Therefore, treatment is aimed at preventing febrile UTI to preserve renal function and avoid the development of reflux nephropathy. This chapter addresses the aspects regarding the evaluation, diagnosis and management of VUR.

Historical Perspective

In the medieval era, Galen and da Vinci were the first to recognize that the ureterovesical junction permitted unidirectional flow of urine from the kidneys into the bladder.[1,2] In 1893, Pozzi reported the existence of VUR in humans, as he once noted a leak of urine from an accidental cut on the distal ureter during a gynecological surgery.[3] He then raised the possibility that VUR might be an abnormal state in humans, although his observations did not allow him to draw conclusions at the time. In 1907, Sampson stated that the oblique course of the ureter through the bladder served as an antireflux mechanism and he associated the presence of VUR and renal infection. [4] One of the most important discoveries related to reflux came from Hutch's classic studies on paraplegic patients (1952), which enabled him to establish a causal relationship between VUR and chronic pyelonephritis. [5] Based on Hutch's observations, Hodson (1959) later revealed that UTI and renal scarring also occurred more often in children with VUR. [6,7] The modern era of VUR was ushered in by Ransley and Risdon's studies (1979), which established the relationship between reflux, infection and renal scarring, therefore outlining the pathophysiology of reflux nephropathy. [4] The clinical studies of Smellie and colleagues (1991) further improved our understanding of the concepts of VUR, bacterial pyelonephritis and renal scarring. [4] Nevertheless, in the last decades, the basis of the medical and surgical management of reflux has been debated among the medical community, moving from a surgical to a more conservative approach. The effectiveness of antimicrobial prophylaxis in preventing recurrences of pyelonephritis and renal damage in children with VUR is a controversial issue, with recent studies showing conflicting results. [8-12] Furthermore, the advent and perfection of new techniques, such as the endoscopic treatment of reflux, may soon reshape our approach to VUR and its treatment indications.

Demographics

The true prevalence of VUR among the general population is hard to define, since the evaluation and diagnosis of reflux is often performed only in symptomatic patients. Nevertheless, it is estimated that VUR affects up to 0.4-1.8% of the pediatric population. [13] A meta-analysis of studies on children undergoing cystography for diverse indications showed a prevalence of VUR in 30% of patients with UTI and up to 17% in patients without infection. [14] In fact, reflux seems to be more common in patients with UTI, occurring in 71% of children younger than 1 year of age, 25% of children at 4 years of age, 15% of children at 12 years of age and 5.2% of adults. [15] The high rate of spontaneous resolution in children leads to the assumption that the incidence of VUR is lower in post-pubertal patients than in infants with febrile UTI. [16,17] Indeed, studies showed that the prevalence of VUR in adult patients is 2.3% to 9%. [16] Moreover, even if reflux is a well-known risk factor for recurrent febrile UTIs in the pediatric population, it is hardly recognized in post-pubertal patients presenting the same findings. In post-pubertal patients, VUR may present as recurrent episodes of UTI, hypertension, renal calculi, back pain or they may even be asymptomatic. [18] Still, VUR must be considered in adult patients, as well as children, who suffer from recurrent bouts of pyelonephritis.

VUR can also be discovered in an asymptomatic patient following the diagnosis of prenatal hydronephrosis. Although fetal hydronephrosis is quite common and often resolves in the neonatal period, studies showed that a diagnosis of reflux is made in up to 15% of infants with absent or mild hydronephrosis on postnatal ultrasound and in 38% of infants with anomalies such as hydronephrosis, renal cysts or renal agenesis. [18,19] In contrast, other studies proposed a prevalence of VUR of 25% in infants undergoing postnatal evaluation of fetal hydronephrosis. [19,20]

There is a higher proportion of males in patients who received a diagnosis of reflux after investigating antenatal hydronephrosis. [21] Ring et al. (1993) showed a preponderance of 76% of male refluxing infants among patients evaluated for VUR after fetal upper tract dilatation. [22] Moreover, boys are more likely to present at younger age and with severe grades of reflux, but they tend to have higher rates of resolution. [23-26] A higher incidence of VUR in young males could be explained by high voiding pressures and small vesical capacity, which affect more boys than girls. [27] Later in life, the majority of patients diagnosed with VUR after an episode of UTI are females, [21] who account for 85% of prevailing reflux in older children. [28] Gender predisposition for VUR may be explained by the incidence of UTI in males and females at a certain age. In fact, a higher incidence of UTI among males or females leads to a greater rate of diagnosis of VUR in this particular population, since they tend to undergo voiding cystourethrogram more often.

Studies showed that VUR is ten times more frequent among female children of Caucasian origin then it is in African girls, and that reflux has a propensity to resolve sooner in the latter population. [29,30] Askari and Belman (1982) showed that among African American children evaluated for UTI, VUR was only one-third as frequent as in white children presenting with the same clinical findings. In this study, however, VUR's evolution after diagnosis was similar in African American and white patients. [31] Nevertheless, after 10 years of age, the incidence of VUR becomes similar between children of all races, raising the hypothesis of differences in the maturation of antireflux mechanisms in patients of African and Caucasian descent. [32] However, many questions remain on the racial predisposition for VUR, due to the fact that the accessible data on reflux come from studies mostly conducted in western and northern European countries.

Genetics

Over the past decades, many authors reported a higher incidence of VUR in siblings and parents of index patients with reflux. In fact, in identical twins, the prevalence of reflux might be as high as 100%,[33] whereas in siblings it is estimated to be around 32-50%.[34-37] Furthermore, high incidence of parent-to-child transmission has been reported, with 66% of affected parents' children having VUR. [38] In regard to these data, various authors proposed that VUR might be an inherited condition with an autosomal dominant pattern and variable penetrance. The hypothesis of a polygenic or multifactorial mode of inheritance has been favored by some authors considering the wide variability of reflux in siblings and published evidences of genetic heterogeneity. [39,40] Indeed, number of loci have been associated with VUR, but no definite etiologic link has been made between these loci and reflux. [40,41]

Many animal studies observed the implication of several genes in the development of the ureteral bud and the integrity of the ureterovesical junction. For instance, the transcription factor PAX2 and the Gdnf RET signaling complex have been associated with the development of the ureteric budding and the ureterovesical junction formation in mice. [42,43] However, none have been shown to be an important factor in the genesis of VUR in humans. [44-46] VUR was also observed in animal models after depletion of the uroplakin III gene, but these observations were not consistent with the findings in human cohorts. [47-49] Genes regulating the renin-angiotensin complex have also been studied, but no strong association with VUR has been discovered. [50] A recent study by Yang et al. on French-Canadian VUR patients reported that 83 out of 118 patients had a rare A allele of SNP rs1799939 and the Gly691Ser mutation, which might interfere with ureteral development. [51] Although the actual studies have not yet been able to identify a genetic pattern for VUR, its high incidence among siblings and parents of affected children might point to a more complex polygenic or multifactorial mode of inheritance.

The Ureterovesical Junction

The peristaltic activity of the ureter propels the urinary bolus towards the UVJ, which is designed to enable the passage of urine into the bladder and to prevent retrograde flow from the compliant bladder to the ureter and renal pelvis. In order to prevent VUR, the intravesical portion of the ureter must first penetrate the bladder wall obliquely. Then, an adequate length of ureter must progress through the submucosal layer of the bladder to finally form a normal shaped ureteric orifice with an appropriate position on the trigone.

Increasing the volume of the bladder during the filling phase creates a flap-valve mechanism by compressing the ureter's intramural and submucosal segments against the detrusor muscle. This antireflux compression valve prevents retrograde flow of urine towards the ureter. In addition, the inherent muscle tone of the intramural ureter creates a moderate obstacle to the passage of urine, allowing only the peristaltic propulsion of urinary bolus from the kidneys.

Appropriate length and obliquity of the intravesical ureter are essential in order to maintain a well functioning UVJ during bladder distension and micturition. Trigonal function represents an important aspect of this antireflux mechanism, as an increase in bladder pressure will stimulate its tone and provide adequate anchoring of the ureteric orifices. In fact, trigonal incompetency is known to be associated with VUR, as it often results in poor anchoring and lateral displacement of the orifices during bladder filling and micturition, which leads to a decrease in the intravesical ureter's length and the effect of the flap-valve mechanism.

Anatomic variations in the shape and location of the orifices are also associated with reflux. Indeed, studies showed a correlation between VUR and lateral positioning or abnormal morphology of the ureteric orifices, which probably results in deficient trigonal anchoring and a shorter intravesical ureter. [52]

Primary and Secondary Vesicoureteral Reflux

In patients presenting with VUR, a distinction can be made between primary and secondary reflux. Primary reflux refers to a congenital deficiency of the ureterovesical junction (UVJ), therefore altering the function of the antireflux mechanism. In primary reflux, bladder dynamics are normal and VUR occurs despite normal intravesical pressures during the storage and voiding phases. In contrast, secondary reflux involves a normal UVJ whose function is impaired due to congenital or acquired bladder anomalies, such as neurogenic bladder disorders or bladder outlet obstruction.

Functional or anatomical bladder obstruction is often the root of elevated voiding pressures, as well as increased muscular tone and storage pressure, which lead to malfunction of the antireflux flap-valve mechanism, therefore causing VUR. The most common example of bladder outlet obstruction occurs in posterior urethral valves (PUV), which are associated with reflux in 48-70% of affected patients. [53-56] Studies showed that relief of obstruction by valve ablation leads to VUR resolution in 78% of patients, therefore pointing to obstruction and elevated intravesical pressures as the cause of secondary reflux. [56]

Neurogenic bladder disorders also predispose to chronic elevation of intravesical pressures, often causing alterations in the bladder wall and secondary dysfunction of the UVJ. In fact, patients with myelodysplasia and untreated neurogenic bladders have an 80% incidence of reflux when bladder pressures exceed 40 cmH_2O. [57,58]

Urodynamic anomalies like detrusor overactivity, obstructive or inadequate voiding patterns in infants have also been associated with VUR. [59] Dysfunctional elimination syndrome and detrusor-sphincter dyssynergia contribute to high voiding pressures and may induce secondary VUR in children. In neurologically intact children, inhibited detrusor contraction is a known cause of secondary reflux and a perpetuating factor for primary reflux. [60-62]

Although primary and secondary reflux are two separate entities, the distinction between both forms is sometimes hard to make, as they may coexist in certain patients. As a matter of fact, bladder dysfunction may be combined to primary reflux, therefore conducting to the aggravation of the UVJ's elemental structural and functional defect.

Classification of Reflux

Many grading and classification systems for VUR have been elaborated throughout the years. In 1981, the International Reflux Study Committee created a five grades scale of reflux, which is based on the anatomy of the ureter, renal pelvis and calyces during the voiding cystourethrogram (VCUG) (Figure 1 and Table 1). The International Classification of Vesicoureteral Reflux is still currently used by clinicians in the diagnosis, the management and follow-up of patients with VUR. However, many factors can influence the degree of VUR seen on the VCUG. For instance, studies showed that bladder dynamics, bladder outlet and ipsilateral UVJ obstruction might modulate the interpretation of the VCUG and the actual grade of reflux. [63] Moreover, in a follow-up perspective, parameters such as bladder dynamics or filling and voiding cycles during the cystogram cannot be perfectly reproduced from one assessment to another. In a given patient, it is safe to assume that a disparity of at least one grade of reflux could be observed between different VCUG studies. A recent study by O'Neil et al. showed high level agreement between raters for grade 1 (0.98) and grade 5 (0.72) reflux, whereas scoring discrepancies were more common for grades 2-4. [64] Radiologists tend to grade VUR higher than urologists and were more likely to differ by more than one grade upon VCUG reading. [64] Therefore, although a grading system is an essential tool for the evaluation of a patient with VUR, clinical judgment must be used in interpreting the results.

Natural History

In patients affected by VUR, the main health concern is the occurrence of pyelonephritis, which can lead to serious consequences such as renal scarring, hypertension and renal insufficiency. In fact, in the presence of bacteriuria, reflux will enable the ascension of microorganisms to the upper urinary tract and the renal parenchyma, therefore promoting the emergence of pyelonephritis. In the same manner, VUR can cause dilatation of the upper urinary tract, creating a reservoir effect for microorganisms and allowing cyclic reintroduction of infected urine from the upper tract to the bladder and from the bladder to the kidneys. Risk factors for bladder colonization also play a role in the individual propensity for pyelonephritis in patients with reflux. Indeed, components such as hygiene and bowel habits can affect the number of organisms that have potential access to the urinary tract. Furthermore, residual urine after bladder emptying or prolonged time between voids are two important factors that influence bacterial incubation in the bladder.

As mentioned previously, VUR facilitates the occurrence of infectious pyelonephritis, and therefore it is associated with the occurrence of renal scarring. The risk for postpyelonephritic scarring is age-related; children younger than one year of age are the most vulnerable to scarring[65] along with patients who present with a febrile UTI whitin the first 4 years of life. [66] Still, acquired renal scarring can develop beyond 5 years of age in children who are not properly treated or suffer from late diagnosis. [67] In newborns with antenatal diagnosed VUR, high grade reflux is sometimes associated with renal maldevelopment, called dysplasia, congenital reflux nephropathy or hypoplasia, which can be difficult to differentiate from postinfection pyelonephritic scars. In fact, studies showed that patients with VUR, particularly of higher grades, can present with findings such as a smaller ipsilateral kidney or reduced renal function[68,69] and that 30-35% of patients will have kidneys that are diminutive or dysmorphic even though they are infection free. [20,70-71]

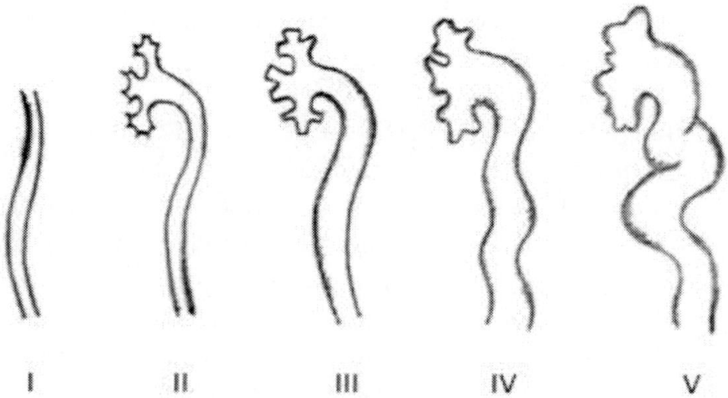

Figure 1. International classification of vesicoureteral reflux.

Table 1. International Grades of Vesicoureteral Reflux

Grade
1 Reflux into a nondilated ureter
2 Reflux reaches the pelvis and calyces, no dilatation of the collecting system
3 Mild to moderate dilatation of the ureter, renal pelvis and calyces with minimally deformed fornices
4 Moderate ureteral tortuosity with dilatation of the collecting system
5 Gross dilatation of the ureter and collecting system, tortuosity of the ureter and loss of papillary impressions

Many studies showed an association between reflux and hypertension in adulthood. [72,73] In fact, patients with renal scarring are known to have a higher risk of developing hypertension, [74] whereas the risk of becoming hypertensive in patients without renal scarring is probably similar to the risk among the normal population. In patients with scarred kidneys, correction or spontaneous resolution of VUR does not alter the risk of developing hypertension, underlining the importance of the management of UTI in the reflux population. [74] Moreover, a greater incidence of hypertension was reported in pregnant women with a history of VUR and renal scarring, with as high as 31% and 42% of pregnancies upon studies. [75] Nonetheless, the higher risk of hypertension in this population was only reported in nulliparous pregnancies. In two studies, pre-eclampsia was documented in 14% and 10% of pregnant women with a history of renal scarring, compared with 1.4% and 2% in the control groups. [75] Among pregnant patients who had undergone ureteric reimplantation, pre-eclampsia was reported in 24% of women, which represents a significant increase compared to the incidence of pre-eclampsia in the general population (0.8-7%). [75]

Renal failure is also a serious consequence of VUR and renal scarring. In fact, reflux nephropathy was once identified as the fourth most common diagnosis in nonblack pediatric transplant patients with end-stage renal disease. [4] Approximately 29% of children presenting with severe reflux and dysmorphic kidneys will suffer from renal insufficiency, proteinuria or hypertension. [76] Moreover, since renal function is known to play a role in somatic growth, patients with VUR often fall in the lower percentiles of the normal growth curve and tend to have inferior weight than children among the normal population. [77,78] Management of recurrent UTIs with either medical or surgical approach in children with reflux can lead to an improvement in both height and weight curves. [78,79] Unfortunately, despite all the progress in the medical field, the number of pediatric patients with reflux nephropathy on the waiting list for kidney transplantation has changed little. In Australia and New Zealand, reflux nephropathy was the second most common diagnosis (19%) in patients with end-stage renal disease and renal replacement therapy. [80] In North America, United States, Japan and Netherlands, the incidence of VUR as primary renal disease in patients with end-stage renal disease varied from 3-7%. [80] In the 2006 Annual Report of the North American Pediatric Renal Trials and Collaborative Studies, reflux nephropathy still was the fourth most common etiology of end-stage renal disease. [81]

VUR has a high rate of spontaneous resolution over time, particularly in younger patients with low-grade reflux. Indeed, it is believed that as children grow older, the intramural ureter lengthens, therefore reshaping the UVJ and improving the antireflux mechanism. In addition, bladder growth and bladder maturation provide better compliance and capacity, leading to an improvement in urodynamics. The American Urological Association (AUA) Vesicoureteral Reflux Practice Guidelines Committee reported a spontaneous resolution rate of 92% of grade 1 and 81% of grade 2 reflux at 5 years of age. Among children with grade 3 VUR, there is a 12,5% to 70% resolution rate depending on age at presentation and the existence of unilateral or bilateral disease. In grade 4 unilateral reflux, 58% of patients will experience spontaneous resolution, whereas 10% of bilateral grade 4 VUR will resolve. [82] Another study reported that high grade reflux resolved or improved in 59% of patients and showed normal renal growth with expectant management in those patients. [83] Older children with persistent reflux are less likely to experience spontaneous resolution [84] perhaps because the anatomical remodelling of the UVJ and bladder growth is completed around age 5. Recently, Cooper et al. (2011) showed an association between the distal ureteral diameter ratio (UDR) and the clinical outcomes of either surgical correction or spontaneous resolution of reflux. In this small series of patients, UDR was found to be more predictive of clinical outcome than the grade of VUR. [85] This parameter could be an additional tool in helping physicians predicting when and in which children VUR is more likely to resolve spontaneously. Likewise, Méndez et al. (2005) documented a relationship between ureteral dilatation and the success rate of endoscopic treatment. [86]

Evaluation of Reflux

The diagnosis of VUR implies the detection of retrograde flow of urine from the bladder to the kidneys. With this in mind, the voiding cystourethrogram (VCUG) represents the present-day gold standard in the evaluation of reflux. After urethral catheterization, contrast is instilled in the bladder and VUR is demonstrated by the ascension of contrast through the ureters to the kidneys. VCUG provides not only information on the dynamics of the urinary tract, but also on its anatomy, showing dilatation of the ureters, renal pelvis or calyces encountered in the different grades of reflux. VUR may be demonstrated during filling or active voiding of the bladder. In a small number of patients, reflux may be observed during catheter filling when bladder pressure is at its lowest, which raises the possibility of a more severe UVJ dysfunction and poorer prognostic. Although there is a general consensus concerning the risk of iatrogenic pyelonephritis in patients undergoing VCUG during an acute UTI, some children with recurrent pyelonephritis and negative cystographies may benefit from a voiding study during active infection. In fact, edema and inflammation associated to UTI may alter the antireflux mechanism of a normally well functioning UVJ in sterile urine. Guidelines recommend the use of oral prophylactic antibiotics for patients undergoing a VCUG in the evaluation of VUR, as urethral catheterization could facilitate the spread of UTI. [87] While VCUG is known to be the gold standard in the evaluation and grading of reflux, exposure to radiations and the need for urethral catheterization are often seen as two major negative aspects of this approach by the patient's family. The radiation dose associated with pediatric VCUG examinations is between 0.1 and 0.5 mSv, [88] compared to 0.02 mSv for a chest x-ray and 1 to 10 mSv for CT imaging. [89] Moreover, positioning and immobilization of the patient, particularly in young children, may be a challenge in performing the VCUG.

Another form of cystography, called a direct radionuclide cystogram (RNC), is performed by filling the bladder with contrast material (usually Technetium Tc99 pertechnetate) and evaluating the presence of VUR with scintigraphic gamma camera images. Radiation exposure from RNC represents approximately 1% of the radiation generated by a VCUG study. [4] Even though RNC allows little anatomical details, it has a higher sensitivity for detecting grade 2 to 5 reflux in relation to its ability to perform continuous imaging. However, RNC shows poor sensitivity for grade 1 VUR because of inadequate visualisation of reflux in the distal ureter due to the overlying exposure of the bladder. Bladder catherization and positioning of the patient remain a challenge in the RNC as well as in the VCUG study. Nevertheless, it can be used in association with VCUG imaging in order to decrease the radiation exposure and still be able to benefit from the dynamic information and anatomical details provide by the VCUG.

Direct magnetic resonance voiding cystourethrography (D-MRVCUG) is a new and promising approach for the evaluation of VUR. This technique showed a sensitivity of 96.8% and a specificity of 96.3% for the evaluation of reflux, when compared to traditional VCUG. [90] Johnin et al. (2013) reported a 96.6% rate of agreement between VCUG and D-MRVCUG regarding the diagnosis of VUR, with D-MRVCUG failing to detect only one case of grade 1 reflux in this study. [90] The main advantage of D-MRVCUG resides in the absence of radiation exposure, which could be a concern in children, especially in patients who undergo repeted VCUGs. On the other hand, this technique presents important limitations, such as the need for complete immobilisation, which can require sedation, and its much higher cost when compared to VCUG. [90]

As mentioned earlier, VUR's effect on renal growth and function are well known. Therefore, renal imaging in patients with reflux is of the highest importance. Ultrasonography is considered the mainstay in documenting the baseline renal dimensions and monitor growth over time. High grades of reflux can present with a loss of the corticomedullary differentiation and increased echogenicity, which are linked to a decreased in renal function. Furthermore, sonography is a valuable tool to assess ureteral dilatation and hydronephrosis. Renal anomalies found upon follow-up ultrasonography in patients with VUR may commend further evaluation of renal function by scintigraphy or the reassessment of the management approach.

Renal scintigraphy (DMSA) is the gold standard in the evaluation of renal function and scar detection. DMSA can be used for the assessment of renal damage in patients whose reflux or infection history is unknown, as well as in patients presenting with an unclear diagnosis of pyelonephritis during an acute episode of UTI. Cortical defects seen upon renal scintigraphy may also help to identify patients who are more likely to develop hypertension or progress towards end-stage renal disease, as there is a correlation between renal scarring and renal function. Furthermore, a decreased renal function on DMSA often commands a more aggressive treatment of VUR or the need of nephrectomy in cases where a surgical management is considered.

The 2007 guidelines from the National Institute for Health and Care Excellence (NICE) represent a useful tool in the assessment of children presenting with urinary tract infection. It details the preferred investigations and management options depending upon patient's characteristics and situation. [87]

Associated Anomalies

Ureteropelvic Junction Obstruction

VUR and ureteropelvic junction obstruction (UPJO) are part of the most common conditions encountered in pediatric urology. Indeed, UPJO is found in 0,75% to 3.6% of patients with a diagnosis of reflux and is five times more frequent with high grades VUR. [91,92] Primary UPJO, which is considered as a true anatomical obstruction, often coexists with reflux, as it is speculated that the UJV and ureteropelvic junction (UPJ) might share the same embryological origin. Secondary UPJO is more likely to be associated with high grades VUR, as it represents a direct result of the dilatation and tortuosity of the urinary tract associated with reflux. In fact, deformation of the proximal ureter along with the decreased contractility of the distended renal pelvis will obstruct the passage of urine through the UPJ in patients suffering from severe VUR. Patients with reflux and UPJO may present with specific patterns upon VCUG. In fact, elements such as the blockage of contrast material at the UPJ and the presence of a dilated and tortuous ureter with a cut-off of contrast at the UPJ suggest a diagnosis of UPJO, as well as a discrepancy in the small calibre of the refluxing ureter and a large renal pelvis. [92] Contrast remaining in the renal pelvis after the ureter and bladder are empty is also an indicator of obstruction. [92] VUR patients whose VCUG show a dilution of contrast material as it enters the renal pelvis and slow drainage of refluxed contrast should be evaluated for UPJO with a Lasix-renogram scan. [93] When both conditions coexist, correction of the UPJO by pyeloplasty must be performed first in order to preserve renal function, since obstruction is more damaging to the kidneys than sterile reflux. However, since secondary UPJO's etiology is linked to VUR, it is speculated that correction of reflux could improve the tortuosity and kinking of the ureter, and therefore obstruction would likely resolve spontaneously. Kajbafzadeh et al. (2013) treated patients suffering from concomitant VUR and UPJO with endoscopic treatment of VUR alone, and achieved a 76.9% and 84.6% rate of spontaneous resolution of the obstruction after the first and second injection respectively. [93]

Duplication

VUR is also one of the most common pathology associated with ureteral duplication in the literature. The correlation between reflux and complete ureteral duplication can be attributed to the lateral insertion of the lower pole ureter and its shorter intravesical segment, which might interfere with the antireflux mechanism of the UVJ. A more aggressive management of reflux has been advocated for these patients in the last decade, as data demonstrated a tendency for VUR to last longer in patients with ureteral duplication and a relationship between high-grade VUR in females and infection and renal scarring. [94,95]

Bladder Diverticulum

Bladder diverticulums, also called Hutch diverticulum, are associated with both primary and secondary VUR. Most commonly, a paraureteral diverticulum predisposes to primary reflux by remodelling the UVJ's structure, thereby altering the normal functioning of the antireflux mechanism. In some cases, a large paraureteral diverticulum can cause ureteral or bladder outlet obstruction, leading to secondary reflux. However, studies showed similar spontaneous resolution rates between patients with reflux and bladder diverticulum and patients with reflux alone, as well as equivalent infection and renal scarring rates. [95]

Multicystic Dysplastic Kidney

Since both UVJ and kidneys share the same embryologic origin, renal anomalies often coexist with VUR. Multicystic dysplastic kidney (MCDK) is associated with a 26% prevalence of contralateral reflux, [96] while 28% of patients with renal agenesis suffer from contralateral VUR. [97] Diagnosis of these conditions used to mandate a VCUG evaluation, since reflux may affect the contralateral compensatory renal hypertrophy in patients with MCDK and show lower rates of spontaneous resolution in patients with renal agenesis. [98,99] However, Miller et al. (2004) reported no significant differences in contralateral renal length in patients with or without VUR and suggested that VCUG could be delayed for 2-3 years since the majority of patients will present with low to moderate grades of VUR and experience high rates of spontaneous resolution. [96] Kuwertz-Broeking et al. (2003) documented low rates of VUR in patients with MCDK and stated that routine VCUG was unnecessary if contralateral upper urinary tract and kidney were normal on ultrasonography. [100] The Canadian Urological Association (CUA) guidelines state that the decision to perform a VCUG study should take into consideration the risks of the child having VUR or developing UTI and/or end-stage renal disease. Children with contralateral hydronephrosis or complex MCDK (bilateral dysplasia or abnormalities of the contralateral kidney or genitourinary tract) detected on ultrasound are at higher risk for reflux, UTI and chronic renal insufficiency. [101]

Surgical Indications for Reflux

Surgical repair is commonly offered to patients who suffer from breakthrough UTIs despite the use of prophylactic antibiotics. Surgery can also be seen as a reasonable option in high grade persistent reflux, particularly in bilateral VUR. It can also be considered in patients with poor compliance to non-surgical treatment or those with little access to health services, and in the case of unreliable parents or parents demanding for a surgical approach.

Traditionally, antireflux surgery was also offered to adolescents and adults who are diagnosed with VUR and experience nonobstructive flank pain or febrile UTIs, since literature showed that reflux persisting throughout teenage years and adulthood is unlikely to resolve spontaneously. [102]

Moreover, the majority of girls with persistent VUR after puberty will undergo corrective surgery, as reflux in adult females carries an increased propensity for maternal and fetal morbidity during pregnancy. In fact, decreased bladder tone and physiologic dilatation of the urinary tract occurring throughout gestation predispose women to bacteriuria, while VUR increases the risk of developing pyelonephritis. Indeed, many studies showed higher rates of infection related complications in pregnant women with hypertension or renal failure or with uncorrected reflux. [4] A review of the literature by Hollowell (2008) reported that the principal factor associated with morbidity during pregnancy was renal scarring, and that women with normal kidneys were not at higher risk for gestational hypertension, pre-eclampsia or fetal morbidity despite persistence of VUR. [75]

Management of Vesicoureteral Reflux

Management of VUR is based on 5 principles, which can be used to guide physicians and patients in their choice of treatment:

1. Majority of children will experience spontaneous resolution of reflux;
2. High grade VUR and reflux in adolescence or adulthood is less likely to disappear spontaneously;
3. Sterile reflux is not associated to renal damage;
4. Antibacterial prophylaxis is safe; and
5. Surgical management has high success rates.

Treatment options can be divided in nonsurgical and surgical management. Conservative therapy is based on two principal approaches: watchful waiting and antibiotic prophylaxis. Surgical management of VUR can be done either with endoscopic treatment or open/laparoscopic/robotic surgical techniques.

Observation

When VUR is diagnosed, physician can attempt to use a watchful waiting approach. If the patient and his or her family choose this option, it is essential to counsel the patient about management of UTI risk factors. In order to prevent infections, patients should first maintain proper genital and perineal hygiene. Children experiencing bladder dysfunction, such as obstructive or inadequate voiding patterns, should go through bladder retraining in order to ensure regular and complete emptying of the bladder and low-pressure voiding. Biofeedback has proven to be an effective therapy for bladder dysfunction, as it enables patients to gain better awareness and voluntary control over pelvic floor muscles during voiding. [103] Maintaining a good level of hydration is also a key element in preventing UTI in children with bladder dysfunction, as it stimulates more frequent micturition and bladder emptying. Good bowel habits and elimination of constipation is also an important aspect of UTI prevention, as constipation is known to reduce micturition volumes, therefore increasing postvoid residual urine, and to induce colonisation of the perineum with pathogens. Moreover, literature showed that anticholinergic treatment of patients with overactive bladder and VUR led to higher spontaneous resolution rates of reflux. [60,62] As a matter of fact, treatment of bladder and bowel dysfunction (BBD) is essential in patients with VUR, as children experiencing BBD have a lower spontaneous VUR resolution rate, a higher risk of UTI and a decreased rate of successful correction of reflux after surgery. [103,104]

Antibiotic Prophylaxis

Traditionally, medical approach to VUR was considered as the first line of treatment for most patients, as reflux tend to resolve spontaneously. Daily low dose of antimicrobial prophylaxis is used in order to maintain sterile urine and prevent febrile UTIs and renal scarring. Recent studies showed conflicting evidence on the effectiveness of antibiotic prophylaxis for the prevention of UTI. In the RIVUR study, prophylaxis reduced the risk of febrile or symptomatic UTI recurrence by 50% compared to placebo. [10] On the other hand, Pennesi et al. reported a lack of effectiveness for long-term antibiotic prophylaxis in preventing pyelonephritis recurrences. [9] However, occurrence of renal scarring were similar among prophylaxis and placebo groups for both studies. [9,10] Conway et al. also came to the conclusion that antimicrobial prophylaxis was not associated with decreased risk of recurrent UTI. [12] Moreover, they reported a higher risk of antimicrobial resistance among children on prophylaxis experiencing recurrent UTI. [12] Other studies showed the benefit of long-term antibiotics in reducing repeated symptomatic UTI and a significant reduction of urinary tract infection in boys taking prophylaxis. [8,11] Still, the American Urological Association and the European Association of Urology guidelines consider the use of antimicrobial prophylaxis as a viable option for initial therapy in the majority of children. [105,106]

Typical antibiotics include trimethoprim, trimethoprim-sulfamethoxazole (TMP-SMX), amoxicillin and nitrofurantoin. TMP-SMX should not be prescribed in children younger than 2 months of age because of hepatic immaturity. Antimicrobial prophylaxis should be given at night time in the toilet trained children, allowing higher concentrations of antibiotic in urine when patients experience physiologic retention and are prone to infections. Although the use of prophylactic antibiotics is considered safe and well tolerated by most patients, side effects can occur. TMP-SMX is known to cause gastro-intestinal upset, allergic reactions, photosensitivity or leucopenia. Nitrofurantoin can produce gastric upset, nausea and has a very poor taste. Discontinuation of antibioprophylaxis was traditionally done as the child approached the age of 5, based on the hypothesis that pyelonephritis in older children is less likely to cause renal damage. Currently, prophylaxis is stopped as soon as VUR's resolution is documented or after acquisition of toilet training to decrease the duration of prophylaxis. Patients on antimicrobial prophylaxis can suffer from breakthrough UTIs, in which cases patient's compliance to treatment must be evaluated, as well as antibiotic dosage. Usually, an episode of breakthrough infection, particularly a febrile UTI, is considered as a failure of non-surgical management and commands consideration of a surgical correction.

Endoscopic Treatment

Endoscopic subureteral injection has gained popularity since its initial description by Matouschek in 1981. [107] In the literature, the use of injections of Teflon for the treatment of reflux in patients was described as early as 1984. [108] For years, ureteroneocystostomy has been the surgical gold standard treatment for patients with VUR. However, controversy remains about the role of endoscopic injection therapy. It is well known that endoscopic treatment of VUR must be individualized. With the arrival of endoscopy, many variables other than VUR grade are now considered in the decision to treat a patient with VUR. Patients' age, sex, history of urinary tract infections, renal status, social status, patients' preferences and the chance and the timing of spontaneous resolution of VUR must be considered. [109] Although not as effective as ureteral reimplantation, endoscopic treatment of VUR has many advantages: high success rates, day surgery, absence of significant postoperative complications, safety of injectable materials and low cost. [16] Few contra-indications to endoscopic injection are reported. Voiding dysfunction is a relative contra-indication to surgical treatment because treatment failure and recurrent urinary tract infections are frequent. [110] High-risk groups like grade 5 VUR, duplicated systems or previous treatment failures are now considered eligible to endoscopic management, but they may have a lower expected response rate. [111] Even in adults, endoscopic management has been described as an effective treatment. [102]

Several bulking agents have been described in the endoscopic treatment of VUR. Many characteristics are sough in an ideal bulking agent: biocompatible, nontoxic, non-migratory, non-antigenic, as well as causing minimal inflammation and preserving its shape and volume. The first bulking agent that popularized the endoscopic treatment of VUR was polytetrafluoroethylene (Teflon). Many studies showed good success rates with Teflon. [108-115] However, it has never obtained its FDA approval secondary to concerns regarding the migration of Teflon paste in different organs following its injection. [116] Because of these safety concerns, the use of Teflon paste as a bulking agent in the bladder is scarce. Cross-linked bovine collagen was then studied for its use in VUR treatment. Large clinical series have reported variable success rates and high relapse rates. [117,118] For these reasons, cross-linked collagen in endoscopic management of VUR has been abandoned by many centers. Thereafter, autologous materiel as blood, chondrocytes, fat and myoblasts were experimented. They seemed to be ideal agents because of their availability and great compatibility. However, fat and chondrocytes showed high rates of long-term failure. [119-121] On the other hand, blood has not been largely studied and the experimental use of myoblasts in pigs failed. [122,123]

The two actual most popular agents in the literature are polydimethylsiloxane (Macroplastique™) and dextranomer/hyaluronic acid

(Dx/HA, Deflux™). Deflux is the only FDA-approved bulking for endoscopic injection of VUR. Many groups have compared the results obtained with injection of polydimethylsiloxane vs Dx/HA copolymer for VUR endoscopic treatment. There is no consensus on the best bulking agent. Kim et al. injected a total of 106 ureters (73 patients) and did not find significant difference between the success rates of Macroplastique™ (87%) and Deflux™ (84%). [124] In 2014, Moore et al. have published a series of 399 ureters (275 patients) injected with either Macroplastique™ or Deflux™. [125] They showed a cure rate at 3 months of 90% with Macroplastique™ and 81% with Deflux™, which was statistically significant. Homldahl et al. studied endoscopic treatment of VUR with dextranomer/hyaluronic acid injections and reported spontaneous resolution or downgrading of reflux in most patients treated. Moreover, two years after treatment, they documented a cure rate of 71% of patients in the dextranomer/hyaluronic acid group, compared to 39% and 48% of patients in the antimicrobial prophylaxis and surveillance groups respectively. [126] A meta-analysis by Elder et al. reported high rates of success with endoscopic treatment (with polytetrafluoroethylene, collagen, dextranomer/hyaluronic acid, polydimethylsiloxane, chondrocytes, or blood), but success rates were lower with higher grades of VUR. In fact, reflux resolution rate was 78,5% for grade 1 and 2, 72% for grade 3, 63% for grade 4 and 51% for grade 5. [127] Furthermore, resolution rates were similar in children and adults, whereas patients with duplicated system or neuropathic bladder showed decreased success rates. [127]

Two new agents have been introduced recently. Polyacrylate polyalcohol (Vantris) has shown a high success rate but the cost effectiveness of the procedure and the high rate of ureteral obstruction necessitate longer follow-up and more clinical data to recommend the use of this bulking agent. [128,129] Polyacrylamide hydrogel (Bulkamid) was first described in 2013 and since today, only one published work on the used of Bulkamid in the endoscopic treatment is available and show promising results. [130] More trials are also needed for this agent prior to extensive use.

Endoscopic injection of VUR is generally performed as a day surgery with the patient under general anesthesia. A cystoscopy is first performed with the patient in lithotomy position. The technique of injection was first called STING for subureteral Teflon injection. The bulking agent is injected into the detrusor muscle immediately beneath the ureteral orifice. In the 2000s, two new injection techniques have been described: the hydrodistention technique (HIT) and the double hydrodistention technique (double-HIT). [131,132] With the HIT, the ureter is distended with irrigation fluid from the cystoscope and the injection is made within the ureteral orifice, beneath the mucosa. Similarly, with the double-HIT technique, the ureter is distended with irrigation fluid but two injections are performed. A first injection is performed more proximally, within the ureteral tunnel, and a second injection more distally, just under the ureteral orifice. Kirsch et al. reported superior success rates with the modified sting procedure (92%) compared to the standard sting approach. [132]

When endoscopic treatment of VUR is considered, the overall rate and morbidity associated with the procedure have to be well understood. As open ureteral reimplantation, contralateral VUR can occur. The rate of contralateral VUR is 5-18% in open series and 4.5-7% after endoscopic treatment. [133] The rate of major complications is low. Obstruction is one of the most common complications reported in the literature with endoscopic injection. Obstruction is often transient, but sometimes may need a ureteral catheter or an open procedure. Moreover, urinary tract infection and bleeding can occur. Voiding dysfunction can be transient after the surgery, secondary to bladder and urethra manipulations. Concerns with the risk of bladder calcification with Macroplastique™ or Deflux™ exposure from bladder mucosa necrosis or erosion have been raised by some authors, suggesting that physicians may need to provide longer follow-up periods to patients. [125]

Patients' follow-up usually includes an ultrasound in the following weeks and a voiding cystouretrography is typically performed at 3 months. If a second injection is needed, a repeat injection can be considered 6 months after the initial one. [4] A maximum of 2 endoscopic treatment of VUR on a same ureter is generally recommended. However, up to three injections have been reported. [134] Open surgery is recommended after multiple failures. Fears regarding future interventions following endoscopic injection have been raised in the literature. Endoscopic injection of VUR does not appear to have a significant technical impact on a future ureteral reimplantation. [135]

Ureteral Reimplantation

The first report of ureteroneocystostomy is credited to Tauffer in 1877 by Bovee in a review article in 1900. [136] In 1952, successful correction of VUR in paraplegic patients was described by Hutch. [137] Since then, multiples techniques for open surgical repair of VUR have been described, modified and translated to laparoscopic techniques. Today, most surgeons employ only a handful of the previously described repairs. However, their application has dramatically changed with the introduction of endoscopic treatment for VUR. [138] Landmark refinements of Hutch's initial operation included the transvesical advancement technique (Politano-Leadbetter) [139], Paquin, [140] Lich-Grégoir, [141,142] the distal tunnel advancement (Glenn-Anderson) [143] and the transtrigonal technique (Cohen). [144]

The success of ureteroneocystostomy for the treatment of VUR is based on several principles regardless of the surgical technique employed. The restoration of the deficient flap-valve mechanism involves the general surgical requirements of tissue handling with preservation of tissue vascularisation. Successful VUR surgery includes creation of a sealed tension-free ureteral anastomosis and a submucosal tunnel length five times longer than the diameter of the ureter over a firm backing. Surgeries have been divided between intra and extra-vesical. Traditionally, intravesical repairs are used in cases of bilateral VUR, concomitant Hutch diverticulum, obstructive megaureter or need of ureteral tailoring. Most popular intravesical repairs includes: Politano-Leadbetter surgery, Cohen's cross-trigonal technique, Glenn-Anderson surgery and Gil-Vernet repair [145]. They are used in regard to ureteral position, size of the distal ureter, bladder thickness and surgeon's preference. Extravesical technique is better known as Lich-Grégoir repair.

The surgical procedure can also be classified based on the position of the submucosal tunnel in relation to the original hiatus, either suprahiatal or infrahiatal. The Politano-Leadbetter and Paquin techniques are described as suprahiatal repair as the goal is to bring the new hiatus above its original insertion. The tunnel in the Politano-Leadbetter repair is directed toward the trigone medial to the original orifice permitting creation of a long tunnel, especially in case of large ureter. Paquin's reimplantation combined the extravesical dissection and creation of the new hiatus and the intravesical anastomosis. The techniques described by Glenn-Anderson and Cohen are classified as infrahiatal tunnel. In the Glenn-Anderson repair the ureter is advanced toward the bladder neck to elongate the submucosal passage of the ureter, which limits the length of the ureteral tunnel. Cohen's technique overcomes these limitations by directing the tunnel across the trigone especially in small and thick bladder. However, subsequent ureteral canulation of the orifices is difficult.

Transperitoneal laparoscopic extravesical reimplantation has been embraced by several groups and seems to give benefits especially in the adolescent and adult population. Success and complication rates seem to approach numbers obtained with open techniques. [146] However, transvesical laparoscopic reimplantation is more challenging with long operative time due to intracorporal suturing, ureteral tunnelling in small working space, demanding learning curve and difficulty to obtain secure closure at the bladder wall level at the time of port removal. [147] Robotic assistance also makes this demanding procedure more efficient, but still not widely practiced. [148,149]

Standard postsurgical management includes renal ultrasound within the first few weeks to assess for the presence of hydronephrosis. Transient, mild hydronephrosis is often described and usually resolved. [150] Bladder and bowel emptying should also be reviewed at each visit and aggressively addressed. Routine VCUG after a simple reimplantation is usually not performed as success rate is high. VCUG should be reserve to patient with postoperative febrile urinary tract infection and persistent hydronephrosis. [150-152] The AUA Pediatric Vesicoureteral Reflux Guidelines Panel published in 1997 an overall success rate of 95.9% in 8061 open ureteral reimplantation in patients with non-dilating VUR. [74] Long-term efficacy is also sustained. [153,154]

Postoperative complications are rare following ureteral reimplantation. Ureteral obstruction has an occurrence rate of around 1%. [149,150,155] Initial management generally implies an indwelling stent or percutaneous nephrostomy tube in the hope that the obstruction is associated to oedema and will resolve. However, a repeat reimplant might be necessary when obstruction is secondary to kinking or stenosis of the ureter. Failure to correct VUR is also rare and most often happens in patients with severe VUR with dilated urinary tract and non-optimal voiding mechanisms. Patience can be necessary after failed ureteral reimplantation as delayed resolution has been documented in a median of 20.4 months. [156] De novo contralateral VUR can also be documented (1-18%) if VCUG is performed in the postoperative period. Contralateral VUR is usually low grade and resolves spontaneously. [157-159] Transient and prolonged urinary retention and voiding dysfunction may present after ureteral reimplantation. [160] Traditionally, these problems have been related to bilateral extravesical ureteral reimplantation but can also be encounter with unilateral technique as the nerves to the bladder run from the pelvis plexus in close proximity to the ureterovesical junction. Finally, subsequent ureteral catheterisation can be more challenging after ureteral reimplantation especially if Cohen's transtrigonal technique was performed.

Open, laparoscopic or robotic ureteral reimplantation still has an important place in the management of VUR. The long term durability of ureteroneocystostomy is excellent with low morbidity.

Conclusion

VUR is one of the most common pathology encountered in pediatric urology. The principal health concern in patients with reflux is the occurrence of pyelonephritis, which can lead to serious consequences such as renal scarring, hypertension and renal insufficiency. The diagnosis of VUR must be considered in adult patients, as well as children, who suffer from recurrent bouts of pyelonephritis. Several management options exist, but the treatment must be tailored to each patient individually, taking into account their age, grade and evolution of reflux, as well as its high rate of spontaneous resolution.

References

[1] Lines, D. 15th century ureteric reflux. *Lancet*, 1982, 2, 1473.

[2] Polk, HC; Jr. Notes on Galenic urology. *Urol Surv*, 1965, 15, 2-6.

[3] Pozzi S. Ureteroverletzung bet laparotomic. *Zentribl Gynacol*, 1893, 17, 97.

[4] Wein, AJ; Kavoussi, LR; Novick, AC. Campbell-Walsh Urology. 10th Edition. Saint-Louis: Saunders, 2011.

[5] Hutch, JA; Miller, ER; Hinman, F Jr. Vesicoureteral reflux. Role in pyelonephritis. *Am J Med*, 1963, 34, 338-49.

[6] Hodson, CJ; Edwards, D. Chronic pyelonephritis and vesico-ureteric reflex. *Clin Radiol*, 1960, 11, 219-31.

[7] Hodson, CJ. The radiology of chronic pyelonephritis. *Postgrad Med J*, 1965, 41, 477-80.

[8] Williams, G; Craig, JC. (2011). Long term antibiotics for preventing recurrent urinary tract infection in children (Review). The Cochrane Library [On-line serial], Issue 3. http,//www.thecochranelibrary.com

[9] Pennesi, M; Travan, L; Peratoner, L; et al. Is Antibiotic prophylaxis in children with vesicoureteral reflux effective in preventing pyelonephritis and renal scars? A Randomized, Controlled Trial. *Pediatrics*, 2008, 121(6), 1489-94.

[10] Hoberman, A; Greenfield, SP; Mattoo, TK; et al. (2014). Antimicrobial prophylaxis for children with vesicoureteral reflux. *The New England Journal of Medecine [On-line serial]*, nejm.org

[11] Roussey-Kesler, G; Gadjos, V; Idres, N; et al. Antibiotic prophylaxis for the prevention of recurrent urinary tract infection in children with low grade vesicoureteral reflux: results from a prospective randomized study. *The Journal of Urology*, 2008, 179, 674-79.

[12] Conway, PH; Cnaan, A; Zaoutis, T; et al. Recurrent Urinary Tract Infections in Children. *JAMA*, 2007, 298(2), 179-86.

[13] Docimo, SG. Kelalis-King-Belman textbook of clinical pediatric urology. 5th Edition. New York: CRC Press, 2007.

[14] Sargent, MA. What is the normal prevalence of VUR? *Pediatr Radiol*, 2000, 30, 587-93.

[15] Baker, R; Maxted, W; Maylath, J; et al. Relation of age, sex, and infection to reflux: data indicating high spontaneous cure rate in pediatric patients. *J Urol*, 1966, 95, 27.

[16] Zilberman, DE; Mor, Y. Has the data Efflux Regarding the Promising Outcome Following Injection of Deflux Changed the Management of Adult Vesicoureteral Reflux? *Advances in urology*, 2008.

[17] Austin, JC. Treatment of Vesicoureteral Reflux after Puberty. *Advances in urology*, 2008, 590185 5 pages.

[18] Phan, V; Traubici, J; Hershenfield, B; et al. Vesicoureteral reflux in infants with isolated antenatal hydronephrosis. *Pediatr Nephrol*, 2003, 18, 1224-8.

[19] Zerin, JM; Ritchey, ML; Chang, AC. Incidental vesicoureteral reflux in neonates with antenatally detected hydronephrosis and other renal abnormalities. *Radiology*, 1993, 187, 157-60.

[20] Burge, DM; Griffiths, MD; Malone, PS; et al. Fetal vesicoureteral reflux, outcome following conservative postnatal management. *J Urol*, 1992, 148, 1743-5.

[21] Yeung, CK; Godley, ML; Dhillon, HK; et al.. The characteristics of primary vesico-ureteric reflux in male and female infants with pre-natal hydronephrosis. *Br J Urol*, 1997, 80, 319-27.

[22] Ring, E; Petritsch, P; Riccabona, M; et al. Primary vesicoureteral reflux in infants with a dilated fetal urinary tract. *Eur J Pediatr*, 1993, 152, 523-5.

[23] Hannula, A; Venhola, M; Renko, M; et al. Vesicoureteral reflux in children with suspected and proven urinary tract infection. *Pediatr Nephrol*, 2010, 25, 1463-9.

[24] Menezes, M; Puri, P. Familial vesicoureteral reflux-is screening beneficial? *J Urol*, 2009, 182(Suppl 4), 1673-7.

[25] Alsaywid, BS; Saleh, H; Deshpande, A; et al. High grade primary vesicoureteral reflux in boys, long-term results of a prospective cohort study. *J Urol*, 2010, 184, 1598-603.

[26] Noe, HN. The long-term results of prospective sibling reflux screening. *J Urol*, 1992, 148, 1739-42.

[27] Sillen, U; Hellstrom, AL; Hermanson, G; et al. Comparison of urodynamic and free voiding pattern in infants with dilating reflux. *J Urol*, 1999, 161, 1928-33.

[28] Shopfner, CE. Modern concepts of lower urinary tract obstruction in pediatric patients. *Pediatrics*, 1970, 45, 194-6.

[29] Skoog, SJ; Belman, AB. Primary vesicoureteral reflux in the black child. *Pediatrics*, 1991, 87, 538-43.

[30] Chand, DH; Rhoades, T; Poe, SA; et al. Incidence and severity of vesicoureteral reflux in children related to age, gender, race and diagnosis. *J Urol*, 2003, 170, 1548-50.

[31] Askari, A; Belman, AB. Vesicoureteral reflux in black girls. *J Urol*, 1982, 127, 747.

[32] Melhem, RE; Harpen, MD. Ethnic factors in the variability of primary vesicoureteral reflux with age. *Pediatr Radiol*, 1997, 27, 750-1.

[33] Kaefer, M; Curran, M; Treves, ST; et al. Sibling vesicoureteral reflux in multiple gestation births. *Pediatrics*, 2000, 105, 800-4.

[34] Hollowell, JG; Greenfield, SP. Screening siblings for vesicoureteral reflux. *J Urol*, 2002, 168, 2138-41.

[35] Kenda, RB; Fettich, JJ. Vesicoureteric reflux and renal scars in asymptomatic siblings of children with reflux. *Arch Dis Child*, 1992, 67, 506-8.

[36] Jerkins, GR; Noe, HN. Familial vesicoureteral reflux, a prospective study. *J Urol*, 1982, 128, 774-8.

[37] Wan, J; Greenfield, SP; Ng, M; et al. Sibling reflux, a dual center retrospective study. *J Urol*, 1996, 156, 677-9.

[38] Noe, HN; Wyatt, RJ; Poeden, JN Jr.; et al. The transmission of vesicoureteral reflux from parent to child. J Urol, 1992, 148, 1869-71.

[39] Burger, RH; Burger, SE. Genetic determination of urologic disease. *Urol Clin North Am*, 1974, 1, 419.

[40] Feather, SA; Malcom, S; Woolf, AS; et al. Primary, non-syndromic vesicoureteric reflux and its nephropathy is genetically heterogeneous, with a locus on chromosome 1. *Am J Human Genet*, 2000, 66, 1420-5.

[41] Chapman, CJ; Bailey, RR; Janus, ED; et al. Vesicoureteric reflux, segregation analysis. *Am J Med Genet*, 1985, 20, 577-84.

[42] Keller, SA; Jones, JM; Boyle, A; et al. Kidney and retinal defects, a transgene-induced mutation with a deletion of mouse chromosome 19 that includes Pax2 locus. *Genomics*, 1994, 23, 309-20.

[43] Yu, OH; Murawski, IJ; Myburgh, DB; et al. Overexpression of RET leads to vesicoureteric reflux in mice. *Am J Physiol Renal Physiol*, 2004, 287, F1123-30.

[44] Choi, KL; McNoe, LA; French, MC; et al. Absence of PAX2 gene mutations in patients with primary familial vesicoureteric reflux. *J Med Genet*, 1998, 35, 338-9.

[45] Cunliffe, HE; McNoe, LA; Ward, TA; et al. The prevalence of PAX2 mutations in patients with isolated colobomas or colobomas associated with urogenital anomalies. *J Med Genet*, 1998, 35, 806-12.

[46] Shefelbine, SE; Khorana, S; Schultz, PN; et al. Mutational analysis of the GDNF/RET-GDNFR alpha signaling complex in a kindred with vesicoureteral reflux. *Hum Genet*, 1998, 102, 474-8.

[47] Hu, P; Deng, FM; Liang, FX; et al. Ablation of uroplakin III gene results in small urothelial plaques, urothelial leakage, and vesicoureteral reflux. *J Cell Biol*, 2000, 151, 961-72.

[48] Giltay, JC; van, de, Meerakker, J; van Amstel, HK; et al. No pathogenic mutations in the uroplakin III gene of 25 patients with primary vesicoureteral reflux. *J Urol*, 2004, 171, 931-2.

[49] Jiang, S; Gitlin, J; Deng, FM; et al. Lack of major involvement of human uroplakin genes in vesicoureteral reflux, implications for disease heterogeneity. *Kidney Int*, 2004, 66, 10-19.

[50] Liu, KP; Lin, CY; Chen, HJ; et al. Renin-angiotensin system polymorphisms in Taiwanese primary vesicoureteral reflux. *Pediatr Nephrol*, 2004, 19, 594-601.

[51] Yang, Y; Houle, AM; Letendre, Julien; et al. RET Gly691Ser Mutation is associated with primary vesicoureteral reflux in the French-Canadian population from Quebec. *Human mutation*, 2008, 29(5), 695-702.

[52] Heale, WF. Age of presentation and pathogenesis of reflux nephropathy. In: Hodson CJ, Kincaid-Smith P, eds. Reflux Nephropathy. New York: Masson, 1979, 140-6.

[53] Reuter, KL; Lebowitz, RL. Massive vesicoureteral reflux mimicking posterior urethral valves in a fetus. *J Clin Ultrasound*, 1985, 13, 584-7.

[54] Puri, P; Kumar, R. Endoscopic correction of vesicoureteral reflux secondary to posterior urethral valves. *J Urol*, 1996, 156, 680-2.

[55] Hassan, JM; Pope, JC; Brock, JW; et al. Vesicoureteral reflux in patients with posterior urethral valves. *J Urol*, 2003, 170, 1677-80.

[56] Priti, K; Rao, KLN; Menon, P; et al. Posterior urethral valves, incidence and progress of vesicoureteric reflux after primary fulguration. *Pediatr Surg Int*, 2004, 20, 136-9.

[57] Flood, HD; Ritchey, ML; Bloom, DA; et al. Outcome of reflux in children with myelodysplasia managed by bladder pressure monitoring. *J Urol*, 1994, 152, 1574-7.

[58] McGuire, EJ; Woodside, JR; Borden, TA; et al. Prognostic value of urodynamic testing in myelodysplastic patients. *J Urol*, 1981, 126, 205-9.

[59] Yeung, CK; Godley, ML; Dhillon, HK; et al. Urodynamic patterns in infants with normal lower urinary tracts or primary vesico-ureteric reflux. *Br J Urol*, 1998, 81, 461-7.

[60] Koff, SA; Murtagh, DS. The uninhibited bladder in children, effect of treatment on recurrence of urinary infection and on vesicoureteral reflux resolution. *J Urol*, 1983, 130, 1138-41.

[61] Homsy, YL; Nsouli, I; Hamburger, B; et al. Effects of oxybutynin on vesicoureteral reflux in children. *J Urol*, 1985, 134, 1168-71.

[62] Seruca, H. Vesicoureteral reflux and voiding dysfunction, a prospective study. *J Urol*, 1989, 142, 494.

[63] Lebowitz, RL. The detection and characterization of vesicoureteral reflux in the child. *J Urol*, 1992, 148, 1640-2.

[64] O'Neil, BB; Cartwright, PC; Maves, C; et al. Reliability of voiding cystourethrogram for the grading of vesicoureteral reflux. *Journal of pediatric urology*, 2014, 10, 107-111.

[65] Winberg, J. Commentary: progressive renal damage from infection with or without reflux. *J Urol*, 1992, 148, 1733.

[66] Smellie, JM; Normand, ICS. Urinary tract infections in children. Postgrad Med, 1985, 61, 895.

[67] Benador, D; Benador, N; Slosman, D; et al. Are younger children at highest risk of renal sequelae after pyelonephritis? *Lancet*, 1997, 349, 17.

[68] Najmaldin, A; Burge, DM; Atwell, JD. Reflux nephropathy secondary to intrauterine vesicoureteric reflux. *J Pediatr Surg*, 1990, 25, 387-90.

[69] Risdon, RA. The small scarred kidney in childhood. *Pediatr Nephrol* 1993, 7(4), 361-4.

[70] Marra, G; Barbieri, G; Moioli, C; et al. Mild fetal hydronephrosis indicating vesicoureteric reflux. *Arch Dis Child Fetal Neonatal Ed*, 1994, 70, F147.

[71] Najmaldin, A; Burge, DM; Atwell, JD. Fetal vesicoureteral relux. *Br J Urol*, 1990, 65, 403.
[72] Barai, S; Bandopadhayaya, GP; Bhowmik, D; et al. Prevalence of vesicoureteral reflux in patients with incidentally diagnosed adult hypertension. *Urology*, 2004, 63, 1045-8, discussion.
[73] Kohler, J; Tencer, J; Thysell, H; et al. Vesicoureteral reflux diagnosed in adulthood. Incidence of urinary tract infections, hypertension, proteinuria, back pain and renal calculi. *Nephrol Dial Transpl*, 1997, 12, 2580-7.
[74] Elder, JS; Peters, CA; Arant, Jr. BS; et al. The pediatric vesicoureteral reflux guideline panel summary report on the management of primary vesicoureteral reflux in children. *J Urol*, 1997, 157, 1846.
[75] Hollowell, JG. Outcome of pregnancy in women with a history of vesico-ureteric reflux. *BJUI*, 2008, 102, 780-4.
[76] Bailey, RR. Sterile reflux, is it harmless? In, Hudson J, Kincaid-Smith P, eds. Reflux Nephropathy. New York: Masson Publishing 1979, 334.
[77] Dwoskin, JY; Perlmutter, AD. Vesicoureteral reflux in children, a computerized review. *J Urol*, 1973, 109, 888.
[78] Polito, C; La, Manna, A; Capacchione, A; et al. Height and weight in children with vesicoureteral reflux and renal scarring. *Pediatr Nephrol*, 1996, 10, 564-7.
[79] Polito, C; Marte, A; Zamparelli, M; et al. Catch-up growth in children with vesico-ureteric reflux. *Pediatr Nephrol*, 1997, 11, 164-8.
[80] Orr, NIT; McDonald, SP; McTaggart, S; et al. Frequency, etiology and treatment of childhood end-stage kidney disease in Australia and New Zealand. *Pediatr Nephrol*, 2009, 24, 1719-1726.
[81] Smith, JM; Stablein, DM; Munoz, R; et al. Contributions of the transplant registry, the 2006 annual report of the north American pediatric renal trials and collaborative studies (NAPRTCS). *Pediatr Transplantation*, 2007, 11, 366-373.
[82] American Urological Association pediatric vesicoureteral reflux clinical guidelines panel. Report on the management of primary reflux in children. Baltimore: American Urological Association, Inc., 1997.
[83] Upadhyay, J; McLorie, GA; Bolduc, S; et al. Natural history of neonatal reflux associated with prenatal hydronephrosis, long-term results of a prospective study. *J Urol*, 2003, 169, 1837-1841.
[84] Skoog, SJ; Belman, AB; Majd, M. A nonsurgical approach to the management of primary vesicoureteral reflux. *J Urol*, 1987, 138, 941-6.

[85] Cooper, CS; Birusingh, KK; Austin, JC; et al. Distal ureteral diameter measurement objectively predicts vesicoureteral reflux outcome. *Journal of pediatric urology*, 2013, 9, 99-103.
[86] Méndez, R; Somoza, I; Tellado, MG; et al. Predictive value of clinical factors for successful endoscopic correction of primary vesicoureteral reflux grades III-IV. *Journal of pediatric urology*, 2006, 2, 545-550.
[87] National Institute for Health and Care Excellence guideline development group. Urinary tract infection in children, diagnosis, treatment and long-term management. Manchester: National Institute for Health and Care Excellence, 2007.
[88] Lee, R; Thomas, KE; Connolly, BE; et al. Effective dose estimation for pediatric voiding cystourethrography using an anthropomorphic phantom set and metol oxide semiconductor field-effect transistor (MOSFET) technology. *Pediatr Radiol*, 2009, 39, 608-615.
[89] U.S. Food and Drug Administration. (2009). Radiation-Emitting Products. FDA [On-line]. http://www.fda.gov/radiation-emitting products/radiationemittingproductsandprocedures/medicalimaging/medicalx-rays/ucm115329.htm
[90] Johnin, K; Takazakura, R; Furukawa, A; et al. Magnetic resonance voiding cystourethrography (MRVCUG): a potential alternative to standard VCUG. *Journal of Magnetic Resonance Imaging,* 2013, 38, 897-904.
[91] Lebowitz, RL; Blickman, JG. The coexistence of ureteropelvic junction obstruction and reflux. *AJR Am J Roentgenol*, 1983, 140, 231-8.
[92] Bomalaski, MD; Hirschl, RB; Bloom, DA. Vesicoureteral reflux and ureteropelvic junction obstruction, association, treatment options and outcome. *J Urol*, 1997, 157, 969-74.
[93] Kajbafzadeh, AM; Tourchi, A; Ebadi, M. The outcome of inital endoscopic treatment in the management of concomitant vesicoureteral reflux and ureteropelvic junction obstruction. *J Urol*, 2013, 81(5), 1040-6.
[94] Estrada, CR; Passerotti, CC; Graham, DA; et al. Nomograms for predicting annual resolution rate of primary vesicoureteral reflux, results from 2,462 children. *J Urol*, 2009, 182, 1535.
[95] Afshar, K. Vesicoureteral reflux and complete ureteral duplication, conservative or surgical management? *J Urol*, 2005, 173, 1725.
[96] Miller, D; Rumohr, J; Dunn, R; et al. What is the fate of the refluxing contralateral kidney in children with multicystic dysplastic kidney? *J Urol*, 2004, 172, 1630-4.

[97] Cascio, S; Paran, S; Puri, P. Associated urological anomalies in children with unilateral renal agenesis. *J Urol*, 1999, 162, 1081-3.

[98] Zerin, JM; Leiser, J. The impact of vesicoureteral reflux on contralateral renal length in infants with multicystic dysplastic kidney. *Pediatr Radiol*, 1998, 28, 683-6.

[99] Song, JT; Ritchey, ML; Zerin, JM; et al. Incidence of vesicoureteral reflux in children with unilateral renal agenesis. *J Urol*, 1995, 153, 1249-51.

[100] Kuwertz-Broeking, E; Brinkmann, OA; Lengerke, HJV; et al. Unilateral multicystic dysplastic kidney: experience in children. *BJUI*, 2004, 93, 388-392.

[101] Psooy, K., Multicystic dysplatic kidney in the neonate: the role of the urologist. *CUAJ*, 2010, 4(2), 95-7.

[102] Moore, K; Bolduc, S. Treatment of vesicoureteral reflux in adults by endoscopic injection. *J Urol*, 2011, 77(6), 1284-7.

[103] Elder, JS; Diaz, M. Vesicoureteral reflux-the role of bladder and bowel dysfunction. *Nat Rev Urol*, 2013, 10, 640-8.

[104] Upahyay, J; Bolduc, S; Bägli, DJ; et al. Use of the dysfunctional voiding symptom score to predict resolution of vesicoureteral reflux in children with voiding dysfunction. *J Urol*, 2003, 169, 1842-1846.

[105] Tekgül, S; Riedmiller, H; Hoebeke, P; et al. EAU guidelines on vesicoureteral reflux in children. *European urology*, 2012, 62, 534-542.

[106] American Urological Association pediatric vesicoureteral reflux clinical guidelines panel. Management and screening of primary vesicoureteral reflux in children: AUA guideline. Baltimore: American Urological Association, Inc., 2010.

[107] Matouschek, E. New concept for the treatment of vesico-ureteral reflux. Endoscopic application of teflon. *Archivos espanoles de urologia*, 1981, 34(5), 385-388.

[108] O'Donnell, B; Puri, P. Treatment of vesicoureteral reflux by endoscopic injection of Teflon. *J Urol*, 2002, 167(4), 1808-9.

[109] Cooper, C. Diagnosis and management of vesicoureteral reflux in children, *Nature reviews urology*, 2009, 6 , 481-489.

[110] Diamond, D; Mattoo, TK. Endoscopic treatment of primary vesicoureteral reflux. *N Engl J Med*, 2012, 366, 1218-26.

[111] Perez-Brayfield, M; Kirsch, AJ; et al., Endoscopic treatment with dextranomer hyaluronic acid for complex cases of vescioureteral reflux. *J Urol*, 2004, 172, 1614-6.

[112] Puri, P. Ten year experience with subureteric Teflon (polytetrafluoro ethylene) injection (Sting) in the treatment of vesicoureteric reflux. *Br J Urol*, 1995, 75 , 126-31.
[113] Hugues, PD. Ureteric reflux in adults and children treated exclusively by endoscopic Teflon injection: a 10-year experience. *Aust NZ J Surg*, 1999, 69, 856-59.
[114] Dewan, P; Higgs, MJ. Correlation of the endoscopic appearance with clinical outcomes for submucous Polytef paste injection in vesico-ureteric reflux. *Aust NZ J Surg*, 1995, 65, 642-4.
[115] Takahide, S; Tadashi, H; et al. Long-term outcome of the endoscopic correction of vesico-ureteric reflux: a comparison of injected substances. *BJUI*, 2004, 94 , 381-83.
[116] Aaronson, IA; Rames, RA; Greene, WE; et al. Endoscopic treatment of reflux, Migration of Teflon to the lungs and brain. *Eur Urol*, 1993, 23, 294-9.
[117] Frey, P; Berger, D; Jenny, P; et al. Subureteral collagen injection for the endoscopic treatment of vesicoureteral reflux in children. Followup study of 97 treated ureters and histological analysis of collagen implants. *J Urol*, 1992, 148 , 718-23.
[118] Stredele, RJF; Dietz, HG; Stehr, M. Long-term results of endoscopic treatment of vesicoureteral reflux in children: Comparison of different bulking agents. *Pediatr Urol*, 2011, 12 , 1-6.
[119] Palma, PCR; Ferreira, U; Ikari, O, et al. Subureteric lipoinjection for vesicoureteral reflux in renal transplant candidates. *Urology*, 1994, 43 , 174-77.
[120] Olson, ME; Morck, DW; Ceri, H ; et al. Evaluation of autologous fat implantation in the rat urinary bladder submucosa. *Urology*, 1998, 52 , 915-19.
[121] Caldamone, AA; Diamond, DA. Long-term results of the endoscopic correction of vesicoureteral reflux in children using autologous chondrocytes. *J Urol*, 2001, 165, 2224-27.
[122] Kohro, K; Kaneko, S; Umekawa, T, et al. Long-term results and curative mechanisms of vesicoureteral reflux by endoscopic injection of blood. *Urology*, 1989, 5, 258-61.
[123] Mitterberger, M; Marksteiner, R; Schwaiger, W ; et al. Can autologous myoblasts be used as a potential bulking agent ? *BJUI*, 2008, 102, 1731-6.
[124] Kim, SO; Shin, BS; Hwang, EC; et al. Clinical efficacy and safety in children with vesicoureteral reflux of a single injection of two diffrent

bulking agents-Polydimethylsiloxane (Macroplastique) or Dextranomer/ Hyaluronic Acid Copolymer (Deflux) , A short-term preospective comparative study. *Urologia int*, 2011, 87 , 299-303.

[125] Moore, K; Bolduc, S. Prospective study of Polydimethylsiloxane vs Hyaluronic acid injection for treatment of vesicoureteral reflux. *J Urol*, 2014, in press.

[126] Holmdhal, G; Brandström, P; Läckgren, G; et al. The Swedish reflux trial in children, II. Vesicoureteral reflux outcome. *J Urol*, 2010, 184, 280-5.

[127] Elder, JS; Diaz, M; Caldamone, AA. Endoscopic therapy for vesicoureteral reflux, A meta-analysis. I. Reflux resolution and urinary tract infection. *J Urol*, 2006, 175, 716-722.

[128] Ormaechea, M; Ruiz, E; Denes, E; et al. New tissue bulking agent (Polyacrylate polyalcohol) for treating vesicoureteral reflux: preliminary results in children. *J Urol*, 2010, 183, 714-18.

[129] Chertin, B; Arafeh, WA; Zeldin, A; et al. Endoscopic correction of VUR using Vantris as a new non-biodegradable tissue augmenting substance, three years of prospective follow-up. *Pediatric urology*, 2013, 82, 201-4.

[130] Cloutier, J; Blais, AS; Moore, K; et al. Prospective study using a new bulking agent for the treatment of vesicoureteral reflux: polyacrylamide hydrogel. *J Urol*, 2013, 190 , 1034-7.

[131] Puri, P; Granata, C. Multicenter survey of endoscopic treatment of vesicoureteral reflux using polytetrafluoroethylene. *J Urol*, 1998, 160 , 1007-1011, 1038.

[132] Kirsch, AJ; Perez-Brayfield, M; Smith, EA; et al. The modified sting procedure to correct vesicoureteral reflux: improved results with submucosal implantation within the intramural ureter. *J Urol*, 2004, 171(6), 2413-6.

[133] Lorenzo, AJ; Khoury, AE. Endoscopic treatment of reflux, management pros and cons, Current opinion. *Urology*, 2006, 16 , 299-304.

[134] Lujan S, Serrano A, Dominguez C, et al. Is a third endoscopic treatment for vesicoureteral reflux indicated if previous attempts have failed? *Pediatr Urol*, 2011, 7 , 650-3.

[135] Moreira-Pinto, J; Osório, A; Pereira, J; et al. Ureteroneocystostomy after failed dextranomer/hyaluronic acid copolymer injection for vesicoureteral reflux treatment. *J Pediatr Urol*, 2013, 9(5), 665-9.

[136] Bovee, JW II. A Critical Survey of Ureteral Implantations. *Ann Surg*, 1900, 32(2), 165-93.

[137] Hutch JA. Vesico-ureteral reflux in the paraplegic, cause and correction. *J Urol*, 1952, 68(2), 457-69.

[138] Herbst, KW; Corbett, ST; Lendvay, TS; Caldamone, AA. Recent trends in the surgical management *J Urol*, 2014, 191(5 Suppl), 1628-33.

[139] Politano, VA; Leadbetter, WF. An operative technique for the correction of vesicoureteral reflux. *J Urol*, 1958, 79(6), 932-41.

[140] Paquin, AJ; Jr. Ureterovesical anastomosis *J Urol*, 1959, 82, 573-83.

[141] Lich, R; Jr. Howerton, LW; Davis, LA. Ureteral reflux, its significance and correction. *South Med J*, 1962, 55, 633-5.

[142] Gregoir, W. The surgical treatment of congenital vesico-ureteral reflux. *Acta Chir Belg*, 1964, 63, 431-9.

[143] Glenn, JF; Anderson, EE. Distal tunnel ureteral reimplantation. *J Urol*, 1967, 97(4), 623-6.

[144] Cohen, SJ. The Cohen reimplantation technique. *Birth Defects Orig Artic Ser*, 1977, 13(5), 391-5.

[145] Gil-Vernet, JM. A new technique for surgical correction of vesicoureteral reflux. *J Urol*, 1984, 131(3), 456-8.

[146] Kasturi, S; Sehgal, SS; Christman, MS; et al. Prospective long-term analysis of nerve *Urology*, 2012, 79(3), 680-3.

[147] Hong, CH; Kim, JH; Jung, HJ; et al. Single-surgeon experience with transvesicoscopic ureteral reimplantation in children *Urology*, 2011, 77(6), 1465-9.

[148] Marchini, GS; Hong, YK; Minnillo, BJ; et al. Robotic assisted laparoscopic ureteral reimplantation in children, case matched comparative study with open surgical approach. *J Urol*, 2011, 185(5), 1870-5.

[149] Song, SH; Kim, KS. Current Status of Robot-Assisted Laparoscopic Surgery in Pediatric Urology. *Korean J Urol*, 2014, 55(8), 499-504.

[150] Grossklaus, DJ; Pope, JC; Adams, MC; et al. Is postoperative cystography necessary after ureteral reimplantation? *Urology*, 2001, 58(6), 1041-5.

[151] Lavine, MA1; Siddiq, FM; Cahn, DJ; Caesar, RE; Koyle, MA; Caldamone, AA. Vesicoureteral reflux after ureteroneocystostomy, indications for postoperative voiding cystography. *Tech Urol*, 2001, 7(1), 50-4.

[152] Barrieras, D; Lapointe, S; Reddy, PP; et al. Are postoperative studies justified after extravescial ureteral reimplantation? *J Urol*, 2000, 164(3), 1064-6.

[153] Hubert, KC; Kokorowski, PJ; Huang, L; et al. Durability of antireflux effect of ureteral reimplantation for primary vesicoureteral reflux, findings on long-term cystography. *Urology*, 2012, 79(3), 675-9.

[154] Garcia-Aparicio, L; Rovira, J; Blazquez-Gomez, E; et al. Randomized clinical trial comparing endoscopic treatment with dextranomer hyaluronic acid copolymer and Cohen's ureteral reimplantation for vesicoureteral reflux: long-term results. *J Pediatr Urol*, 2013, 9(4), 483-7.

[155] Steffens, J; Langen, PH; Haben, B; et al. Politano-leadbetter ureteroneocystostomy. A 30-year experience. *Urol Int*, 2000, 65(1), 9-14.

[156] Hubert, KC; Kokorowski, PJ; Huang, L; et al. Clinical outcomes and long-term resolution *J Urol*, 2012, 188(4 Suppl), 1474-9.

[157] Hubert, KC; Kokorowski, PJ; Huang, L; et al. New contralateral vesicoureteral reflux after unilateral ureteral reimplantation, predictive factors and clinical outcomes. *J Urol*, 2014, 191(2), 451-7.

[158] McCool, AC; Pérez, LM; Joseph, DB. Contralateral vesicoureteral reflux after simple and tapered unilateral ureteroneocystostomy revisited. *J Urol*, 1997, 158(3), 1219-20.

[159] Diamond, DA; Rabinowitz, R; Hoenig, D; et al. The mechanism of new onset contralateral reflux following unilateral ureteroneocystostomy. *J Urol*, 1996, 156(2), 665-7.

[160] Barrieras, D; Lapointe, S; Reddy, PP; et al. Urinary retention after bilateral extravesical ureteral reimplantation, does dissection distal to the ureteral orifice have a role? *J Urol*, 1999, 162(3), 1197-200.

In: Vesicoureteral Reflux and Pyelonephritis ISBN: 978-1-63463-497-7
Editor: Leanna P. Newport

Chapter III

Endoscopic Treatment of Vesicoureteral Reflux

Anne-Sophie Blais, M.D., Stéphane Bolduc, M.D. and Katherine Moore, M.D.
Division of Urology, Department of Surgery,
CHU de Québec, Université Laval, Québec, Canada

Abstract

Management of vesicoureteral reflux has evolved since the 80's, especially due to the introduction of endoscopic approach. Endoscopic treatment of vesicoureteral reflux has gained popularity because of its minimally invasive character and its favorable success rate. It has become an established alternative to antibiotic prophylaxis and invasive surgical intervention. Literature on subureteral endoscopic injection is growing. Many advances in the indications of treatment, composition of bulking agents and injection techniques have emerged in the past decade. Herein, we propose to review indications for endoscopic treatment, technique of injection, different bulking agents and their success rates and finally, adverse events related to their use.

Introduction

Vesicoureteral reflux (VUR) is the result of a short ureteral tunnel combined with the absence of an adequate detrusor support behind the intravesical ureter. It is the most common cause of hypertension in children and young adults [1]. In addition, 5% of patients with end-stage renal disease have reflux nephropathy as their primary diagnosis [1, 2]. The primary goal of VUR treatment is to avoid pyelonephritis and eventually renal scarring, and to preserve renal function. Different management strategies can come into consideration: active surveillance, antibiotic prophylaxis, endoscopic injection or ureteral reimplantation.

Endoscopic subureteral injection has gained popularity and has evolved as a prime therapeutic alternative either from antibiotic prophylaxis or ureteroneocystostomy since its initial description by Matouschek in 1981 [3] and the first clinical series reported by O'Donnell and Puri in 1984 [4]. The ideal bulking agent should be biocompatible, nontoxic, non-migratory, non-antigenic, as well as causing minimal inflammation and preserving its shape and volume. Several types of injectables have been investigated for the treatment of VUR and stress urinary incontinence (SUI), each leading to different safety issues and success rates: polytetrafluoroethylene (PTFE) [4], bovine collagen [5], autologous material (chondrocytes [6], fat [7], blood [8], myoblasts [9]), calcium hydroxyapathite [10], polydimethylsiloxane (Macroplastique™) [11], dextranomer/hyaluronic acid copolymer (Deflux™) [12], polyacrylate polyalcohol (Vantris™) [13] and more recently polyacrylamide hydrogel (Bulkamid™) [14]. The perfect agent is yet to be identified. Herein, we propose to review in this chapter technique of injection, different materials used, success rates and adverse events related to their use.

Surgical Indications

Formal indications for surgical treatment of VUR remain unclear. The goals of VUR management are to prevent febrile urinary tract infection, to prevent renal injury and to minimize morbidity of treatment and follow-up modalities [15]. These goals can be achieved either by conservative treatment, antibiotic prophylaxis or surgical treatment. Traditionally, the decision to undergo a surgical treatment was based on the grade of VUR and age of the patient. Since the last decades, indications of surgery are way less straightforward.

Some physicians recommend surgical management when VUR does not resolve by toilet-training age while others recommend treating surgically patients with severe grade of VUR and pyelonephritis, renal scars and\or related nephropathy [16]. The most common accepted indications for surgery are: breakthrough UTI despite the use of prophylactic antibiotics or surveillance, persistent high-grade reflux particularly if bilateral, symptomatic adults and new renal scars. Moreover, surgical treatment is considered in patients with poor compliance to non-surgical treatment, those with restricted access to health care services and in children who's parents prefer to undergo surgical treatment. Finally, the majority of girls with persistent VUR after puberty will undergo corrective surgery, as reflux in adult females carries an increased propensity for maternal and fetal morbidity during pregnancy [17, 18].

Endoscopic injection therapy for VUR is described as a treatment option by the American Urological Association (AUA) [15]. It is described as a treatment option for children with breakthrough urinary tract infection (UTI) or for children more than 1 year of age with VUR and UTI.

However, despite all the indications described above, recent studies show that VUR management must be individualized [19]. With the arrival of endoscopy and with the best understanding of the physiopathology and natural history of VUR, other variables are now considered in the decision to treat patients with VUR. Patients' age, gender, history of UTIs, renal status, social status, patients' preferences and the probability and the timing of spontaneous resolution of VUR must be considered [19].

Surgical options for VUR correction include endoscopic injection, intra- or extra-vesical ureteral reimplantation, and laparoscopic/robotic reimplantation [20]. Many advantages have been mentioned with regard to endoscopic management in children: good success rates, short or no hospital stay, absence of significant postoperative complications, safety of injectable materials and low cost [21].

Very few contraindications to endoscopic injection are reported. Voiding dysfunction is a relative contraindication to surgical correction because treatment failure and recurrent urinary tract infections are frequent if the voiding dysfunction is not corrected preoperatively [22].

High-risk groups like patients with Hutch diverticula, ureteral duplication, ectopic ureter or prune belly syndrome are now considered available to endoscopic management with a known lower success rate [23]. Even in adults, endoscopic management has been described as an effective treatment [24]. Higher surgical morbidity has been described with ureteral reimplantation in adults secondary to a wider and deeper pelvis post-puberty. However, it should be noted that, in general, ureteral reimplantation has shown better success rates than endoscopic injection [20, 25]. Contrary to popular belief, Garcia-Aparicio et al. reported similar success rates of ureteral reimplantation and endoscopic injection [26]. However, as noted by Canning, low grade of VUR (grade III or less) dominated in this study [27].

Even if a first subureteral injection of bulking agent has failed, a repeat injection can be considered 6 months after the initial one [17]. A maximum of 2 endoscopic treatments of VUR on the same ureter is generally recommended. However, up to three injections have been reported [28]. Ureteral reimplantation is recommended after multiple failures. Fears regarding future interventions following endoscopic injection have been raised in the literature. Endoscopic injection of VUR does not appear to have a significant technical impact on a future ureteral reimplantation [29].

Description of the Different Bulking Agents

Polytetrafluoroethylene (Teflon)

PTFE has been used as a medical device for many years. PTFE is used in gastroenterology for palliative biliary metallic stents, in neurosurgery as artificial dura matter, in thoracic surgery for mitral valve repair and many other properties of PTFE have been described in the literature [30-32]. Teflon paste particles range from 4 to 100 μm, with 90% of the particles being less than 40 μm.

Matouschek first reported Teflon endoscopic injection for the treatment of VUR [3]. PTFE consists of a 50% suspension of polytetrafluoroethylene particles in glycerin. Teflon acts as a foreign body and causes infiltration of histiocytes with a fibrous reaction. In 1995, the management of pediatric VUR with Teflon was popularized by Puri. He reported a series of 258 children treated with injection of Teflon [33]. In 1995, he also published a large European multicenter survey, which included 4166 children for a total of 6216 ureters treated by Teflon injection [33]. The survey demonstrated that 95% of all ureters treated were cured or showed significant improvement after two injections of Teflon. Patients were followed for a period ranging from 3 months to 8.5 years. Many other series were published after Puri's reports and showed high success rates with endoscopic subureteric injection of Teflon [34-36]. A comparative study showed a higher overall success of Teflon over cross-linked bovine dermal collagen, Deflux and autologous blood for endoscopic management of VUR [8]. The overall success rate was the highest at five years with PTFE (63%), followed by 56%, 53% and 8% with collagen, Deflux and autologous blood respectively.

PTFE has been widely used in Europe. However, it has never obtained US Food and Drug Administration approval because of concerns regarding the migration of Teflon particles. Mittleman and Marracini reported a case of multiples pulmonary granulomas composed of Teflon and giant cells in a man who died of suicide and who had received two injections of Teflon for urinary incontinence 1 and 2 years prior to his death [37]. Aaronson et al. also reported migration of Teflon to lung and brain of experimental animals that were given a Teflon injection in the subureteric region [38].

Safety concerns with Teflon paste injection and the availability of many other bulking agents have discouraged the use of Teflon for the endoscopic treatment of VUR.

Cross-Linked Bovine Collagen

The use of cross-linked bovine collagen for the endoscopic treatment of VUR remains a subject of debate. Frey et al. demonstrated a success rate of 77.3% after 2 injections with a mean follow-up of 18.5 months [39]. However, the success rates are widely variable between the different studies. Stredele et al. demonstrated a success rate of 52% at 3 months with a high rate of relapse (48.5%) on long-term follow-up [40].

The hypothesis for the wide range success rate and the high rate of relapse seems to be the variable degree of ingrowth of native fibroblasts and the shrinkage of the bulking agent [41]. Moreover, immunological reactions after collagen injection have been reported. Skin test before the injection is recommended.

Because of the inconsistency of the success rate and the high relapse rate, cross-linked bovine collagen in endoscopic management of VUR has been abandoned by many centers.

Autologous Material

Autologous Chondrocytes

The implantation of autologous chondrocytes was experimented in animal models by Atala and colleagues in the 90's [42]. They were looking for a new injectable material because of concerns related to the long-term safety and effectiveness of collagen and Teflon. They harvested and expanded in vitro cartilage obtained from the auricular surface of 4 mini-pigs. The cells were then injected in the subureteral region. It has been shown to be effective to cure VUR. This experimental work has generated a craze for the procedure. Caldamone et al. published in 2001 a clinical trial using endoscopic injection of autologous chondrocytes in 47 ureters (29 children) [6]. They reported a success rate of 55% (ureters) at 3 months after 1 injection. The success rate was increased to 86% after a second or third injection. Four patients underwent open ureteral reimplantation because of failure of the endoscopic treatment. In all 4 cases, the implant has shifted towards the bladder neck or misplaced deep into the bladder wall. The pathology of the explanted chondrocyte implant revealed calcified alginate without evidence of viable chondrocytes. The authors have extrapolated that the absence of viable chondrocytes was responsible for the treatment failure. They proposed to work on a new formulation to enhance chondrocytes viability. To our knowledge, no other clinical trial has been reported since this publication, more than 10 years ago.

Autologous Fat

Autologous fat was first described as bulking agent for the treatment of urinary incontinence. Initial experiments performed on rats and published reports on periurethral injection for urinary stress incontinence were disappointing [43]. Palma et al. performed lipoinjection of 12 ureters in renal transplant candidates in 1993 [44]. Reduction of grade of reflux was seen in 2 patients. There was no change in the 10 remaining patients. Chancellor et al. also reported 7 patients treated with subtrigonal autologous fat injection [7]. Only 2 patients out of 7 were cured 6 months after the injection. Two of the five remaining patients had a lower grade of VUR. Moreover, the extent and duration of fat graft survival was disappointing. Studies showed that between 10% and 30% of the fat implant survives after injection [45]. Necrosis was responsible for the elimination of the implant. They implanted adipose tissues in the bladder neck mucosa of rats. By day 35, most of the fat was eliminated by phagocytosis. Fat implant is not currently used in the treatment of vesicoureteral reflux.

Autologous Blood

Only few studies reported on the use of autologous blood for the treatment of VUR. Kohri et al. showed in 1988 that submucosal endoscopic injection of blood at the ureteral orifice corrected VUR in dogs [46]. The same group reported in 1989 a series of 13 patients (16 ureters) with low grade VUR, injected with patients' own heparinized blood behind the ureteral orifice [9]. The treatment was successful in 9 of the 16 ureters at 3 months. The treatment was less successful for patients with VUR grade III (1 of 3 ureters). Publications on the use of autologous blood implant remain sparse.

Autologous Myoblasts

Autologous myoblasts have been investigated in pigs to evaluate their potential as an autologous bulking agent [47]. Large bulk of cells could not survived and the vast majority of cells became necrotic. Subureteral injection of myoblasts has never been tried in humans. The use of myoblasts as a bulking agent is not recommended.

Calcium Hydroxyapathite

Calcium hydroxyapatite (CaHa) is a 100 μm particle synthetic agent. Its chemical composition is identical to teeth and bone. It was first used in urology as a bulking agent in the treatment of urinary stress incontinence [48]. The use of CaHa as a new bulking agent in VUR was first investigated in animals. Bakhtiari et al. experimented subureteral injection of calcium hydroxyl apatite in 12 dogs [49]. The total success rate of the injection at 6 months was 91.7%. No migration of the bulking agent was found in other organs and gross examination of the vesicoureteral region showed a sustainable mass of the bulking agent over time.

CaHa was then experimented in humans. Only few studies are available in the literature and success rates reported are widely variable. Tarcan et al. underwent injection of CaHa in 14 patients and showed a success rate of 47.4% after a single injection with a median follow-up of 52 months [10]. One patient underwent a nephroureterectomy due to a non-functioning kidney secondary to ureteral obstruction following injection.

Ngo et al. showed a success rate per ureter of 52% after one injection (voiding cystourethrogram (VCUG) was done 1 to 3 months after the injection) [48]. They compared CaHa with dextranomer hyaluronic acid. When controlling for the learning curve, dextranomer hyaluronic acid appeared to show higher success rates than CaHa. Further studies with bigger cohorts and longer follow-up are needed.

Polydimethylsiloxane (Macroplastique™)

Macroplastique™ has been first commercialized in Europe in 1991 and received Health Canada's approval in 1998. The American Food and Drug Administration have more recently (2006) approved it for the treatment of stress urinary incontinence.

Macroplastique™ is composed of a solid polydimethylsiloxan elastomer (40% of volume) in a bio-excretable hydrogel carrier (non-iodine povidone). It has gained popularity because of its low risk of migration due to its large particle size (median minimum diameter of 140 μm), its composition and its texture [50]. The tissue reaction at the site of injection shows a well-encapsulated foreign body reaction. The carrier gel is absorbed and replaced by giant cells, fibroblasts and collagen deposition [51].

Many urologists have recorded their success rate with subureteral endoscopic injection of Macroplastique™. Herz et al. have shown an overall success rate of 81% after a single injection at an average follow-up of 18 months in 112 ureters [52]. In a selection of 24 studies of sufficient level of evidence, Aubert has performed a literature review on the use of Macroplastique™ in pediatric and adult VUR [53]. He reported an overall success rate at 1 year, 2 years and 9 years follow-up of 86-93%, 80-92% and 77-100% respectively. The success rate was similar for primary and secondary VUR, except for duplicated systems. He mentioned that the higher viscosity and absence of shrinkage of the product increased its reliability.

Endoscopic injection of Macroplastique™ for the treatment of VUR requires specific equipment, including a specific gun to ensure high pressure during the injection. It has been reported that this gun might be difficult to handle for inexperienced people [54].

Dextranomer Hyaluronic Acid (Deflux™)

Deflux™ is a viscous gel consisting of dextranomer microspheres of 80 to 120 μm in diameter and non-animal hyaluronic acid. It is a dextranomer hyaluronic acid copolymer (DxHA) in sodium hyaluronan solution. The product is biocompatible, which means that the material does not cause any significant reaction within the body.

The bulking agent generates an inflammatory reaction with ingrowth of fibroblasts and finally, deposition of autologous collagen [55]. Deflux™ was FDA approved in 2001 for the treatment of VUR. It remains the only FDA approved bulking agent for endoscopic injection of VUR.

Depending on the reflux grade, the overall success rate reported in the literature ranges between 68 and 92% [56]. A systematic review of the published success rates of vesicoureteral injection for pediatric VUR has shown an overall success rate per ureter of 77% at 3 months [57]. Increased VUR grade negatively affected success rates, whereas patient age and volume injected of bulking agent were not associated with treatment outcome.

A German study by Stredele et al. noted a success rate of 81.5% at the initial 3-month post-operative VCUG [40]. However, 21.5% of the patients with initial success relapsed at the 3-year post-operative VCUG. The initial 20% loss of volume within the first 2 weeks following injection seemed to stay relatively stable for at least 3 years (35% loss of volume, $p>0.5$) [58].

Many groups have compared the results obtained with a single injection of polydimethylsiloxane vs DxHA copolymer for VUR endoscopic treatment. Bae et al. reported in 2010 the injection of 115 ureters (71 patients) [59]. They found a cure rate of 80.6% with Macroplastique and 78.6% with Deflux™. No clinically significant differences were found between the 2 groups.

Similarly, Kim et al. injected a total of 106 ureters (73 patients) and did not find a significant difference between the success rates of Macroplastique™ (87%) and Deflux™ (84%) [50].

In 2014, Moore et al. have published a series of 399 ureters (275 patients) injected with either Macroplastique™ or Deflux™ [60]. They showed a cure rate at 3 months of 90% with Macroplastique™ and 81% with Deflux™. The endoscopic injection of polydimethylsiloxane resulted in a significantly higher success rate when compared to hyaluronic acid.

Polyacrylate Polyalcohol Copolymer (Vantris™)

Vantris™ is a biocompatible agent made of microparticles of polyacrylate polyalcohol copolymer (PPC) in glycerol and physiological solution [13]. The majority of the particles have an average diameter of 300µm. Vantris™ has not been investigated only for vesicoureteral reflux, but also for gastro-esophageal reflux, aesthetic surgery, stress urinary incontinence and fecal incontinence. Ormaechea et al. have evaluated in 2008 the properties of Vantris™ in dogs' urethra [61]. They reported that Vantris™ creates a low cellular growth and a low cellular interaction secondary to its high electronegativity. No migration of the agent has been reported. The long-term histology tests showed that the bulking agent was diffusing deeper than the submucosa, which reduce the bulkiness of the agent.

In 2010, Ormaechea et al. described the preliminary results of polyacrylate polyalcohol copolymer in children with VUR [13]. They injected a total of 88 ureters (grade II-V) with a median follow-up of 20 months. A renal and bladder ultrasound and a VCUG were performed at 1-year follow-up. Reflux was cured in 78 renal units (88.6%). One patient experienced ureteral obstruction and underwent an extravesical ureteral reimplantation. Four (6.6%) additional patients developed lumbar pain postoperatively. An editorial comment by Dr. J. Routh mentions that future protocols for PPC injection should consider warning patients that the risk of obstruction may be higher compared to other agent [62]. In 2013, Chertin et al. reported a 3 years follow-up of endoscopic injection of Vantris™ [63]. They injected a total of 165 refluxing renal units (RRU) of grade I to V. An ultrasound was performed at 1 month, 1 year and 3 years after the surgery. A VCUG was also performed at 3 months, 1 year and 3 years. VCUG was performed in 39.1% patients who completed 1 year of follow-up and 40% who completed 3 years of follow-up. VUR was corrected in 92.7% of RRUs after the first injection and this success rate was increased by 4.2% after the second injection. Ureteral obstruction was recorded in 2 patients (1.8%). The ureteral obstruction was treated with insertion of a stent for one patient and ureteral reimplantation for the other.

The results obtained with endoscopic treatment of VUR using Vantris™ appear promising. However, only few published series are available on Vantris™ and cost effectiveness of the bulking agent has been questioned. Also, Dr Routh raised the point that ureteral obstructions are common in many series and are worrisome [62].

More clinical data with longer follow-up seem necessary.

Polyacrylamide Hydrogel (Bulkamid™)

Polyacrylamide hydrogel (PAHG) is a polymer gel consisting of 2.5% cross-linked polyacrylamide and 97.5% water. It is a biocompatible agent, micro-particle-free, non-resorbable and migration-resistant. Bulkamid™ is actually approved as a periurethral bulking agent for female urinary stress incontinence. Its safety and efficacy in urinary incontinence has been documented in previous studies [64-66]. Its efficacy for the treatment of VUR has been recently studied by Cloutier et al. showing a 1-year success rate of 81.2% in 40 patients (69 ureters) [14]. It is the only published report on the used of Bulkamid™ in the endoscopic treatment of VUR. A prospective comparison of Bulkamid™ and Deflux™ is currently in progress. Further trials would be worthwhile to recommend this agent for the endoscopic treatment of VUR.

Injection Technique

The goal of the endoscopic injection of VUR is to create a solid support behind the intravesical ureter without impeding the normal flow of urine from the kidney to the bladder. This support allows elongating the intramural part of the ureter. To achieve a proper endoscopic injection of VUR, many techniques have been described.

Regardless of the injection technique performed, patients with VUR should have an initial evaluation before surgery. The AUA recommends to perform a general medical evaluation (height, weight, blood pressure) and to obtain serum creatinine and urine analysis in children with VUR [15]. Renal ultrasound is recommended at the initial evaluation and DMSA renal imaging can be obtained to assess kidneys' scars and function. Even if there is no recommendation on obtaining a VCUG preoperatively, VCUG is a frequent radiological exam performed preoperatively to assess the grade of reflux. Moreover, urine culture should be done prior to the surgery. A urinary infection must be properly treated before the surgery.

In 1984, the technique of endoscopic injection of bulking agent was first described and was given the acronym STING for subureteral Teflon injection [22]. The term STING is now widely accepted regardless of the bulking agent injected. In North America, the procedure is generally performed as day surgery with the patient under general anesthesia. Cystoscopy is performed with the patient in lithotomy position. An injection needle is placed through the operating channel of the cystoscope. The needle and the syringe can differ depending on the type of bulking agent used for the injection. STING technique consists of the injection of bulking agent into the detrusor muscle immediately beneath the ureteral orifice at the 6 o'clock position (Figure 1). It is advisable to keep the needle in place after the injection for 20-30 seconds to avoid back leaking of the agent [55]. Multiple needle punctures are not recommended for the same reason. The injection of bulking agent with STING technique creates a prominent mound that uplifts the orifice and elongates the intramural ureter.

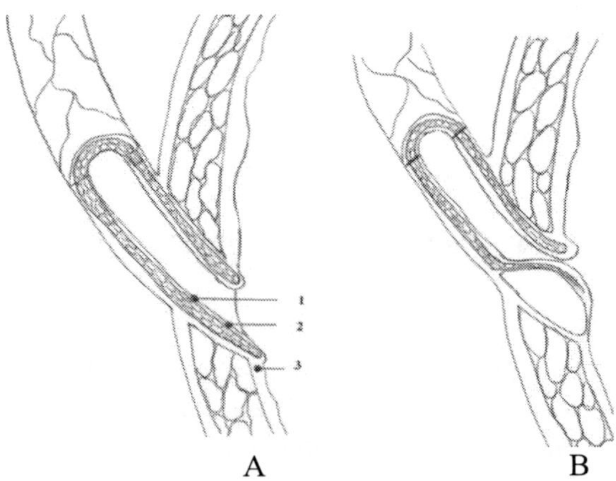

Figure 1. A. Injection sites: 1-2 Double Hit Technique, 3 STING. B. Result post-injection.

Because of a higher success rate with ureteral reimplantation compared to endoscopic injection with the STING technique, a new technique called HIT (hydrodistention implantation technique) has been introduced in 2004 [67]. In this technique, the ureter is distended with irrigation fluid from the cystoscope. The injection is made within the ureteral orifice beneath the mucosa at the 6 o'clock position. This type of injection creates coaptation of the ureteral tunnel by the bulking agent. Improved visualization of the injection site and easier manipulation of the needle were reported with this new technique.

The approach was subsequently modified by the double-HIT technique. This approach consists of two injections. While the ureter is distended with irrigation fluid, a first injection is performed more proximally and a second injection more distally within the ureter (Figure 1). This injection leads to coaptation of the ureteral orifice. Moreover, because the injection is made in the submucosal plane, the length of the ureteral coaptation is maximized.

Following injection with any of the three following techniques, the bladder is emptied. The mound is inspected with an empty and a full bladder. If inadequate support of the ureter is found, another puncture can be done, usually with the STING method. The patients can urinate normally and can continue their activities of daily living after the procedure.

Patients' follow-up usually includes an ultrasound in the following weeks and voiding cystourethrogram is typically performed at 3 months. Antibioprophylaxis is usually continued until the VCUG shows absence of VUR. Persistent VUR following a first injection can be treated with a second injection, usually 6 months after the initial injection [17]. As described above, a third injection can be considered [28]. Ureteral reimplantation is recommended after multiple failures.

Factors Predicting Success of Endoscopic Treatment

Many potential mechanisms of failed endoscopic injection for VUR have been investigated. Many studies have focused on the appearance of the mound, injection technique, surgeon's opinion and experience, grade of reflux, number of injections, bladder and bowel dysfunction, volume of bulking agent injected and complex cases.

Mound Appearance

The goal of the endoscopic injection for the treatment of VUR is to create a mound that elevates and coapts the ureteral orifice. This «mountain-like» appearance of the ureteral tunnel and orifice has been well described by

Molitierno et al. [68]. Yucel et al. have shown in their multivariate analysis that satisfactory mound morphology strongly correlates with good outcomes [69]. A nice appearing implant with an elevated and coapted orifice was achieved in 81% of ureters and reflux resolved in 87% of these ureters. Conversely, a success rate of 36% was described in ureters in which elevation and coaptation of the orifice failed. They indicated that cystoscopic appearance of the implant was the most important factor predicting VUR outcome. Similarly, the appearance of the implants on ultrasound after injection therapy was investigated [70]. The appearance of the mound on postoperative ultrasound showed good correlation with VCUG results. However, the correlation between the perfect mound and the success of the injection therapy is still controversial in the literature. Mound appearance was not a determinant of the success rate in the multi-institutional study done by Higham-Kessier and al. [71]. Many reasons have been raised to explain VUR persistence in spite of good mound morphology. The volume of bulking agent loss 3 months after the injection may cause failure despite appropriate injection [72]. Another reason is that mound morphology may not appropriately indicate the quality of tissue distortion along the intramural ureter. Moreover, mound displacement may be a mechanism of failure.

Injection Technique

The HIT and the double HIT methods were first introduced at the beginning of the 2000s. These two techniques were introduced as a modified STING procedure to improve the success rate of the endoscopic injection of VUR. However, optimal injection technique seems controversial. STING and HIT methods have been compared in different studies. These studies showed non-unanimous results. Routh et al. reported the superiority of HIT over STING technique [73]. However, in their multivariate analysis, this superiority became insignificant. Yucel et al. and Watters et al. found no differences on VUR resolution rate between the 2 techniques [69, 74]. The success rates of HIT and double HIT were also compared. Akin et al. observed a higher success rate with double HIT treatment compared to HIT [75]. The current trend for the preferred injection technique in the United States is the double HIT method [67].

Surgeon's Experience

It is well known that surgeon's experience is one of the most important determinants predicting the success of the endoscopic treatment of VUR [72, 76]. The learning curve is especially important for higher VUR grades. In their series, Kirsch et al. obtained a success rate of 60% within their first 20 patients injected, compared to 80% for their subsequent 20 patients [77]. Of note, both cohorts of patients were comparable for gender, age, grade, bilaterality and volume injected. Dave et al. also strengthened the association of surgeon's experience with successful endoscopic VUR correction [72]. The concept of learning curve is widely used for many other surgical techniques. Endoscopic treatment of VUR does not make exception to this rule.

Preoperative VUR Grade

Many other factors have been identified to have an impact on the success of VUR endoscopic treatment. Many studies agree that lower preoperative VUR grades are predictive of successful VUR correction [69, 72, 74].

Although several studies do not agree on the most important factor predicting the success of the procedure, VUR grade is clearly the most often cited [78].

Repeat Injections

In their literature review, Routh and Reinberg have raised the question of repeat injections: does repeat injection has a lower success rate compared to the first injection? [78] Actual literature does not allow us to answer this question because of lack of comparative data and statistical power in published studies. This lack of data may be due to the small number of patients who undergo a second injection due to the good success rate of the first injection. Some authors recommend up to three injections if the two previous injections failed [28]. According to Lujan, the third treatment has a similar efficacy to the first and second treatment [28].

Bladder and Bowel Dysfunction

In 2010, the AUA Reflux Guidelines Committee performed an analysis of the association of bladder and bowel dysfunction (BBD) [15, 79]. Their meta-analysis showed a lower rate of VUR self-resolution and surgical correction in children with BBD. Children with BBD treated with subureteral injection therapy had a resolution rate at 3-12 months of 50% compared to 89% for those without BBD [79].

Moreover, they reported that children with BBD are at increase risk of UTI before and after surgical correction. Consequently, it has been recommended that toilet training should be encouraged with addition to pharmacological treatment at least 6 months prior to the endoscopic therapy [80]. Moreover, biofeedback may be a good treatment option before surgery. It has proven to be an effective therapy for bladder dysfunction, as it enables patients to gain better awareness and voluntary control over their pelvic floor muscles during voiding. [79]. However, the impact of BBD on the success of the procedure is less clear in other series [78]. This incertitude in the literature may be due to the subjectivity and the variability of the term BBD.

Volume of Bulking Agent

The volume of bulking agent injected to create a mound has also been investigated. However, it remains unclear if it influences the outcome of endoscopic injection. Urologists seem to inject more volume of bulking agent over time [72]. It is believed that a greater volume of bulking agent optimizes the fixation of the implant, prevents its displacement and compensates for the long-term volume loss. Volume loss is of great concern, especially with Deflux™. A 20% relapse rate at 2-years after successful treatment is described with Deflux™ due to its composition compared to Macroplastique™ which is known for its stability over time [40, 81]. Volume loss with the most recent bulking agents as Bulkamid™ and Vantris™ are unknown and longer-term investigations are needed. However, it has also been suggested that a high volume of bulking agent injected may suggest increasing difficulty in achieving the desired mound appearance [69].

Complex Cases

Complex cases of VUR; duplicated systems, post ureterocele incision, grade V VUR and failure after ureteral reimplantation, do not seem to have a lower success rate after endoscopic injection. Chertin et al. injected 37 patients (38 RRU) with complex cases of VUR with Vantris™ [82]. The reflux was corrected in 89.4% of RRU after a single injection at 3 months. Of note, authors have adapted their injection technique according to the anatomy of the patient and its primary pathology. For example, they used the previously described technique of STING for patients with VUR grade I to III. In patients with grades IV and V VUR and in those with a widely open orifice, the injection was performed inside the orifice. Patients with a duplex system were treated with the needle introduced under the bladder mucosa, 2–3 mm below the lower ureteric orifice at the 6 o'clock position. The implant was placed submucosally.

Similarly, Bartoli et al. reported the effectiveness of endoscopic injection of VUR in duplex renal systems [83]. They obtained VUR resolution/ improvement in 88% of patients with duplex system and 95% with single renal system. No statistical significance was reached when comparing both success rates. Perez-Brayfield et al. also reported their experience with children presenting different complicated situations as duplicated system, neurogenic bladder, ectopic ureters and failed open surgery [23]. Good success rates were reported with endoscopic injection procedure.

However, studies comparing patients with primary VUR vs. secondary VUR are lacking.

Moreover, possible complications and benefits of the endoscopic injection of VUR have to be weighted in complex cases. For example, Chertin does not recommended, in light of Snodgrass report, to proceed to an endoscopic injection of refluxing primary megaureter because of the high risk of obstruction [82].

Finally, endoscopic management of VUR in renal transplants has been investigated. Clinical and radiological success rates were poor and widely variable with collagen, Teflon, Macroplastique™ and Deflux™ [84].

Considering all of the above and the possible complications associated with surgery, some authors advocate the use of antibioprophylaxis and surveillance only for these complex cases [85].

Complications

Bleeding

Major bleeding following subureteral injection of bulking agent is rare. When bleeding occurs, it is recommended to empty the bladder and to gently apply the tip of the cystoscope at the bleeding site until the bleeding stops [17]. Cauterizing the bleeding site is not advisable but sometimes necessary if distant from the ureteral orifice. No further treatment is usually required.

Infection

Urinary tract infection is a reported complication following subureteral endoscopic injection. Many patients with VUR have already experienced previous pyelonephritis. Because they are at high risk of recurrence, urine culture must be repeated before the surgery to make sure urines are sterile. Active urinary tract infection is a contraindication to endoscopic injection due to the risk of disseminated infection.

However, even with these precautions, some patients will get infected after the surgery. Heckler et al. reviewed retrospectively 175 patients who underwent endoscopic management of VUR [86]. Most patients had febrile UTIs preoperatively. They reported a 30% incidence of lower urinary tract infection and a 10% of febrile UTI. They did not find any significant correlation between UTI and preoperative patient's characteristics as gender, age, reflux grade, BBD and duplicated system. However, recurrent VUR correlated significantly with both postoperative UTI and febrile UTI. Patients with higher number of preoperative UTIs were also more likely to have postoperative febrile UTIs. On the other hand, Chi et al. studied the incidence of symptomatic UTI after successful correction of VUR with dextranomer/ hyaluronic [87]. Their median follow-up was 42 months. They showed post-injection rate of UTI of 24%. Half of the patients who presented UTI were febrile and half of the patients with febrile UTI had recurrent VUR at the VCUG. They also showed that the number of preoperative urinary tract infections best predicted the likelihood of repeated infection. These two previous series mentioned that their rates of UTI were similar to those reported following ureteral reimplantation.

Kandem et al. showed similar results following injection of DxHA [88]. They showed 18.9% rate of febrile UTI with a median follow-up of 51.6 months. They identified 3 new risk factors for postoperative UTI: cystitis cystica at the time of injection, preoperative renal scarring and disappearance of the implant at 3-month follow-up ultrasound.

Considering all of the above, most series on endoscopic management of VUR recommend to continue antibiotic prophylaxis until the 3-month postoperative VCUG. Febrile UTI following endoscopic injection should be investigated with a VCUG to document VUR recurrence. These investigations should be done even if the injection was made several months or years ago. Voiding habits should also been questioned. A good level of hydration, proper genital and perineal hygiene and elimination of constipation are important aspects of UTI prevention.

Obstruction

Ureteral obstruction is one of the most common complications related in the literature to endoscopic injection. The timing of the obstruction is widely variable, from immediately after the procedure to several months post-operatively. It may manifest by renal colic, hydroureteronephrosis, urinary tract infection or lower urinary tract symptoms. It can also remain asymptomatic and be discovered at the postoperative ultrasound. Because of the potential irreversible renal damages, ureteral obstruction is a worrisome complication. It is assumed that many factors can contribute to the obstruction rate. One of these factors is the choice of the bulking agent. Ureteral obstruction has been reported with most bulking agents. It has been described with polytetrafluoroethylene, polydimethylsiloxane and DxHA [89]. However, the higher rate of obstruction was noted with polyacrylate polyalcohol copolymer. Alizadeh et al. reported a 6% obstruction rate following endoscopic injection of Vantris™ [89]. Excess amount of bulking agent has also been highlighted as a risk factor [90]. However, this correlation is not well described in the literature. Finally, background diseases affecting bladder mucosa as dysfunctional voiding and myelomeningocele, gender and injection technique were reported to have an impact on ureteral obstruction. Literature on these correlations is poor and further evaluation is needed [88].

Many treatments have been described to treat ureteral obstruction following an endoscopic injection of VUR. Ureteral stenting, percutaneous nephrostomy, ureteral reimplantation, balloon dilatation and nephroureterectomy are different treatment options [91-93]. The treatment must be individualized to each patient.

Contralateral Vesicoureteral Reflux

As in open ureteral reimplantation, contralateral VUR can occur after endoscopic injection. The rate of contralateral VUR is 5-18% in open series and 4.5-7% after endoscopic treatment [94]. However, the rate of de novo contralateral VUR seems to be higher in patients treated conservatively rather than surgically. To explain the finding of de novo contralateral reflux after a subureteral endoscopic injection, Kirsch et al. theorized that VUR treatment for the correction of the initial refluxing unit may have created a higher pressure bladder system [77].

Unlike ureteral reimplantation, distortion of the trigone does not occur with injection therapy. Injecting both ureters as a prophylactic treatment is not actually recommended. Contralateral VUR is often of low grade and has no consequence. Moreover, de novo VUR has a high rate of spontaneous resolution over time, particularly in younger patients with low-grade reflux. However, Kirsch et al. proposed that contralateral non-refluxing ureter might be treated when it is abnormally configured (hydrodistension) or located, because of high rates of contralateral reflux and low morbidity of the procedure [77].

Calcification

Implanted agents for endoscopic treatment of VUR have the potential of causing inflammatory and foreign body reactions. Calcification of implants has been reported with many different bulking substances as polytetrafluoroethylene, collagen, autologous chondrocytes, polydimethylsiloxane and DxHA [60, 95]. Symptoms reported with mound calcification are gross or microscopic hematuria with or without intermittent back pain. According to Gargello and al., mound calcification is not a cause of significant morbidity [95]. Treatment of theses calcifications may be needed if symptoms persist. Successful excision of mound calcification with ureteroscopy and biopsy forceps has been reported in a symptomatic 16-year old girl [96]. On the other hand, concerns with the risk of bladder calcification with Macroplastique™ or Deflux™ exposure from bladder mucosa necrosis or erosion have been raised by some authors, suggesting that physicians may need to provide longer follow-up periods after injection [97, 98].

However, the etiology and the impact of these calcifications remain unknown. Indications of treatment are also misunderstood. Urologists must be aware of this possible complication because it may be confused with large distal ureteral lithiasis and lead to unnecessary procedures [99, 100].

Conclusion

Endoscopic subureteral injection has gained popularity and has evolved as primary therapeutic alternative for the treatment of VUR. Despite differences in material proprieties, available bulking agents are safe for the treatment of patients with VUR with few complications.

Several materials have been evaluated with different success rates and adverse events. Recurrence of VUR, febrile UTI, ureteral obstruction and distal calcification are the main concerns after endoscopic injection and should be monitor on the long term. Literature on the endoscopic treatment of VUR is still growing. The future may yield improvements in the technique of injection and the different bulking agents used.

References

[1] Jacobson, S. H., Hansson, S., Jakobsson, B. Vesico-ureteric reflux: occurrence and long-term risks. *Acta paediatrica*, Nov. 1999; 88(431): 22-30.

[2] Pelletier, A. K., Anderson, P. A., Schwarz, R. D. Comparison of different substances for subureteric injection in the management of vesicoureteric reflux in children. *The Canadian journal of urology*, Aug. 2005; 12(4): 2774-2777.

[3] Matouschek, E. [New concept for the treatment of vesico-ureteral reflux, Endoscopic application of teflon]. *Archivos espanoles de urologia*, Sep.-Oct. 1981; 34(5): 385-388.

[4] O'Donnell, B., Puri, P. Treatment of vesicoureteric reflux by endoscopic injection of Teflon, *British Medical Journal*, Jul. 7 1984; 289(6436): 7-9.

[5] Lipsky, H., Wurnschimmel, E. Endoscopic treatment of vesicoureteric reflux with collagen, Five years' experience. *Br. J. Urol.*, Dec. 1993; 72 (6): 965-968.

[6] Caldamone, A. A., Diamond, D. A. Long-term results of the endoscopic correction of vesicoureteral reflux in children using autologous chondrocytes. *J. Urol.*, Jun. 2001; 165(6 Pt 2): 2224-2227.

[7] Chancellor, M. B., Rivas, D. A., Liberman, S. N., et al. Cystoscopic autogenous fat injection treatment of vesicoureteral reflux in spinal cord injury. *The Journal of the American Paraplegia Society,* Apr. 1994; 17 (2): 50-54.

[8] Sugiyama, T., Hanai, T., Hashimoto, K., et al. Long-term outcome of the endoscopic correction of vesico-ureteric reflux: a comparison of injected substances. *BJU Int.*, Aug. 2004; 94(3): 381-383.

[9] Kohri, K., Kaneko, S., Umekawa, T., et al. Long-term results and curative mechanisms of vesicoureteral reflux by endoscopic injection of blood. *Urology*, 1989; XXXIV (5): 258-261.

[10] Tarcan, T., Tinay, I., Temiz, Y. Long-term results of endoscopic treatment of vesicoureteral reflux with the sub-ureteric injection of calcium hydroxyapatite. *International Urology and Nephrology*, Dec. 2007; 39(4): 1011-1014.

[11] Lorenzo, A. J., Pippi Salle, J. L., Barroso, U., et al. What are the most powerful determinants of endoscopic vesicoureteral reflux correction? Multivariate analysis of a single institution experience during 6 years. *J. Urol.*, Oct. 2006; 176(4 Pt 2): 1851-1855.

[12] Stenberg, A., Lackgren, G. A new bioimplant for the endoscopic treatment of vesicoureteral reflux: experimental and short-term clinical results. *J. Urol.*, Aug. 1995; 154(2 Pt 2): 800-803.

[13] Ormaechea, M., Ruiz, E., Denes, E., et al. New tissue bulking agent (polyacrylate polyalcohol) for treating vesicoureteral reflux: preliminary results in children. *J. Urol.,* Feb. 2010; 183(2): 714-717.

[14] Cloutier, J., Blais, A. S., Moore, K., et al. Prospective study using a new bulking agent for the treatment of vesicoureteral reflux: polyacrylamide hydrogel. *J. Urol.*, Sep. 2013; 190(3): 1034-1037.

[15] Peters, C. A., Skoog, S. J., Arant, B. S., et al. Summary of the AUA guideline on management of primary vesicoureteral reflux in children. *J. Urol.*, Sept. 2010; 184: 1134-1144.

[16] Herbst, K. W., Corbett, S. T., Lendvay, T. S., et al. Recent trends in the surgical management of primary vesicoureteral reflux in the era of dextranomer/hyaluronic acid. *J. Urol.*, May 2014; 191: 1628-1633.

[17] Wein, A. J., Kavoussi, L. R., Novick, A. C. *Campbell-Walsh Urology*. 10th Edition, Saint-Louis: Saunders; 2011.

[18] Hollowell, J. G. Outcome of pregnancy in women with a history of vesico-ureteric reflux. *BJUI* 2008; 102: 780-4.

[19] Cooper, C. Diagnosis and management of vesicoureteral reflux in children. *Nature reviews urology*, Sept. 2009; 6: 481-489.

[20] Austin, J. C. Treatment of vesicoureteral reflux after puberty. *Advances in Urology*, 2008: 1-6.

[21] Zilberman, D. E. Has the data efflux regarding the promising outcome following injection of deflux changed the management of adult vesicoureteral reflux? *Advances in urology*, 2008; 1-5.

[22] Diamond, D., Mattoo Tej, K. Endoscopic treatment of primary vesicoureteral reflux. *N. Engl. J. med.*, 2012; 366: 1218-26.

[23] Perez-Brayfield, M., Kirsch, A. J., et al. Endoscopic treatment with dextranomer hyaluronic acid for complex cases of vescioureteral reflux. *J. Urol.*, Oct. 2004; 172: 1614-6.

[24] Moore, K., Bolduc, S. Treatment of vesicoureteral reflux in adults by endoscopic injection. *Urology*, 2011; 77: 1284-87.

[25] Kirsch, A., Hensle, T., Scherz, H., et al. Injection therapy: advancing the treatment of vesicoureteral reflux. *J. Pediatr. Urol.*, 2006; 2: 539-544.

[26] Garcia-Aparicio, L., Rovira, J., Blazquez-Gomez, E. Randomized clinical trial comparing endoscopic treatment with dextranomer hyaluronic acid copolymer and Cohen's ureteral reimplantation for vesicoureteral reflux: long-term results. *J. Pediatr. Urol.*, Aug. 2013; 9 (4): 483-7.

[27] Canning, D. A. Re: Randomized Clinical Trial Comparing Endoscopic Treatment with Dextranomer Hyaluronic Acid Copolymer and Cohen's Ureteral Reimplantation for Vesicoureteral Reflux: Long-Term Results. *J. Urol.*, May 2014; 191(5): 1407-1409.

[28] Lujan, S., Serrano, A., Dominguez, C., et al. Is a third endoscopic treatment for vesicoureteral reflux indicated if previous attempts have failed? *J. Pediatr. Urol.*, Dec. 2011; 7: 650-3.

[29] Moreira-Pinto, J., Osório, A., Pereira, J., et al. Ureteroneocystostomy after failed dextranomer/hyaluronic acid copolymer injection for vesicoureteral reflux treatment. *J. Pediatr. Urol.* 2013; 9(5): 665-9.

[30] Zurstrassen, C. E., Santos, A. C., Tyng, C. J., et al. Percutaneous use of ePTFE/FEP-covered metallic stent for palliation of malignant biliary obstruction. *Minim. Invasive Ther. Allied Technol.*, July 2014; 15: 1-8.

[31] Matsumoto, Y., Aikawa, H., Tsutsumi, M., et al. Histological examination of expanded polytetrafluoroethylene artificial dura mater at 14 years after craniotomy: case report. *Neurol. Med. Chir.* (Tokyo), 2013; 53(1): 43-6.

[32] Ragnarsson, S., Sjögren, J., Sanchez, R., et al. Polytetrafluoroethylene neochordae is noninferior to leaflet resection in repair of isolated posterior mitral leaflet prolapse: a multicentre study. *Interact. Cardiovasc. Thorac. Surg.*, July 2014.

[33] Puri, P. Ten year experience with subureteric Teflon (polytetrafluoro ethylene) injection (Sting) in the treatment of vesicoureteric reflux. *Br. J. Urol.,* 1995; 75: 126-31.

[34] Hugues, P. D. Ureteric reflux in adults and children treated exclusively by endoscopic Teflon injection: a 10-year experience. *Aust. NZ J. Surg.*, 1999; 69: 856-59.

[35] Sauvage, P., Becineur, F., Blentz, J., et al. Endoscopic treatment of vesico-urethral reflux in children with Teflon: A ten year experience. *Br. J. Urol.*, 1997; 2: 170.

[36] Dewan, P., Higgs, M. J. Correlation of the endoscopic appearance with clinical outcomes for submucous Polytef paste injection in vesico-ureteric reflux. *Aust. NZ J. Surg.*, 1995; 65: 642-644.

[37] Mittleman, R. E., Marracini, J. V. Pulmonary Teflon granulomas following periurethral Teflon injection for urinary incontinence. *Arch. Pathol. Lab. Med.,* 1983; 107: 611-612.

[38] Aaronson, I. A., Rames, R. A., Greene, W. E., et al. Endoscopic treatment of reflux: Migration of Teflon to the lungs and brain. *Eur. Urol.*, 1993; 23: 294-9.

[39] Frey, P., Berger, D., Jenny, P., et al. Subureteral collagen injection for the endoscopic treatment of vesicoureteral reflux in children. Followup study of 97 treated ureters and histological analysis of collagen implants. *J. Urol.*, Aug. 1992; 148: 718-23.

[40] Stredele, R. J. F., Dietz, H. G., Stehr, M. Long-term results of endoscopic treatment of vesicoureteral reflux in children: Comparison of different bulking agents. *J. Pediatr. Urol.*, 2011; 12: 1-6.

[41] Frey, J., Chamson, A., Raby, N., et al. Collagen bioassay by the contraction of fibroblast-populated collagen lattices. *Biomaterials*, Jan. 1995; 16(2): 139-43.

[42] Atala, A., Cima, L. G., Kim, W., et al. Injectable alginate seeded with chondrocytes as a potentiel treatment for vesicoureteral reflux. *J. Urol.*, 1993; 150: 745.

[43] Mathews, R. D., Christensen, J. P., Canning, D. A., et al. Persistence of autologous free fat transplant in bladder submucosa of rats. *J. Urol.*, 1994; 152: 819.

[44] Palma, P. C. R., Ferreira, U., Ikari, O., et al. Subureteric lipoinjection for vesicoureteral reflux in renal transplant candidates. *Urology*, 1994; 43: 174-77.

[45] Olson, M. E., Morck, D. W., Ceri, H., et al. Evaluation of autologous fat implantation in the rat urinary bladder submucosa. *Urology*, 1998; 52: 915-19.

[46] Kohri, K., Kataoka, K., Akiyama, T., et al. Treatment of vesicoureteral reflux by endoscopic injection of blood. *Urol. Int.*, 1988; 43(6): 324-6.

[47] Mitterberger, M., Marksteiner, R., Schwaiger, W., et al. Can autologous myoblasts be used as a potential bulking agent? *BJUI*, Dec. 2008; 102: 1731-6.

[48] Ngo, T. C., Wong, I. Y. Z., Kennedy, W. A. A comparison of calcium hydroxyapatite and dextranomer/hyaluronic acid for the endoscopic treatment of vesicoureteral reflux. *Advances in Urology*, 2013; 1-5.

[49] Bakhtiari, J., Kajbafzadeh, A. M., Marjini, M., et al. Endoscopic treatment of vesicoureteral reflux using calcium hydroxyl apatite in dogs. *BMC Research Notes*, 2011; 4: 14.

[50] Kim, S. O., Shin, B. S., Hwang, E. C., et al. Clinical efficacy and safety in children with vesicoureteral reflux of a single injection of two diffrent bulking agents-Polydimethylsiloxane (Macroplastique) or Dextranomer/ Hyaluronic Acid Copolymer (Deflux): A short-term preospective comparative study. *Urologia Int.*, 2011; 87: 299-303.

[51] Choo, M. S., Hong, B., Ji, Y. H., et al. Endoscopic treatment of vesicoureteral reflux with polydimethylsiloxane in adult women. *European Urology*, 2004; 45: 787-789.

[52] Herz, D., Hafez, A., Bagli, D., et al. Efficacy of endoscopic subureteral polydimethylsiloxane injection for treatment of vesicoureteral reflux in children: a North American clinical report. *J. Urol.*, Nov. 2001; 166(5): 1880-6.

[53] Aubert, D. Vesico-ureteric reflux treatment by implant of polydimethylsiloxane (Macroplastique): Review of the litterature. *Prog. Urol.*, Apr. 2010; 20(4): 251-9.

[54] Oswald, J., Riccabona, M., Lusuardi, L., et al. Prospective comparison and 1-year follow-uo of a single endoscopic subureteral polydimethylsiloxane versus dextranomer/hyaluronic acid copolymer injection for treatment of vesicoureteral reflux in children. *Pediatr. Urol.*, 2002; 60(5): 894-898.
[55] Leonard, M. P. Endoscopic injection therapy for treatment of vesicoureteric reflux: a 20-year perspective. *Peadiatr. Child Health*, Oct. 2002; 7(8): 545-550.
[56] Chertin, B., Kocherov, S., Chertin, L., et al. Endoscopic Bulking Materials for the Treatment of Vesicoureteral Reflux: A Review of Our 20 Years of Experience and Review of the Literature. *Advances in Urology*, 2011; 309626.
[57] Routh, J. C., Inman, B. A., Reinberg, Y. Dextranomer/hyaluronic acid for pediatric vesicoureteral reflux: systematic review. *Pediatrics*, May 2010; 125(5): 1010-1019.
[58] McMann, L., Scherz, H., Kirsch, A. Long-term preservation of dextranaomer/hyaluronic acid copolymer implants after endoscopic treatment of vesicoureteral reflux in children: A sonographic volumetric analysis. *J. Urol.* 2007; 177: 316.
[59] Bae, Y. D., Park, M. G., Oh, M. M., et al. Endoscopic Subureteral Injection for the Treatment of Vesicoureteral Reflux in Children: Polydimethylsiloxane (Macroplastique) versus Dextranomer/Hyaluronic Acid Copolymer (Deflux). *Korean J. Urol.*, Feb. 2010; 51(2): 128-131.
[60] Moore, K., Bolduc, S. Prospective study of polydimethylsiloxane vs hyaluronic acid injection for treatment of vesicoureteral reflux. *J. Urol.*, Dec. 2014; in press.
[61] Ormaechea, M., Paladini, M., Pisano, R., et al. Vantris, a biocompatible, synthetic, non-biodegradable, easy-to-inject bulking substance. Evaluation of local tissular reation, localized migration and long-distance migration. *Arch. Esp. Urol.*, 2008; 61(2): 263-268.
[62] Routh, J. Editorial Comment. *J. Urol.*, 2010; 183: 718.
[63] Chertin, B., Arafeh, W. A., Zeldin, A., et al. Endoscopic correction of VUR using Vantris as a new non-biodegradable tissue augmenting substance: three years of prospective follow-up. *Pediatric Urology*, 2013; 82: 201-204.
[64] Christensen, L., Nielsen, J., Mouritsen, L., et al. Tissue Integration of Polyacrylamide Hydrogel: An Experimental Study of Periurethral, Perivesical, and Mammary Gland Tissue in the Pig. *Dermatologic Surgery,* 2008; 34: S68-S77.

[65] Lose, G., Sorensen, H. C., Axelsen, S. M., et al. An open multicenter study of polyacrylamide hydrogel (Bulkamid®) for female stress and mixed urinary incontinence. *Int. Urogynecol. J.,* 2010; 21(12): 1471-7.

[66] Toozs-Hobson, P., Al-Singary, W., Fynes, M., et al. Two-Year follow-up of an open-label multicenter study of polyacrylamide hydrogel (Bulkamid®) for female stress and stress-predominant mixed incontinence. *Int. Urogynecol. J.*, Apr. 2012.

[67] Kirsch, A. J., Arien, A. M., Lackgren, G. Current trends in dextranomer hyaluronic acid copolymer (Deflux) injection technique for endoscopic treatment of vesicoureteral reflux. *Urology*, 2014; 84(2): 462-468.

[68] Molitierno, J. A., Scherz, H. A., Kirsch, A. J. Endoscopic treatment of vesicoureteral reflux using dextranomer hyaluronic acid copolymer. *Pediatr. Urol.*, 2007; 4: 221-228.

[69] Yucel, S., Gupta, A., Snodgrass, W. Multivariate analysis of factors predicting success with dextranomer/hyaluronic acid injection for vesicoureteral reflux. *J. Urol.*, Apr. 2007; 177: 1505-1509.

[70] Park, K. J., Jeon, T. Y., Yoo, S. Y., et al. The appearance of dextranomer-hyaluronic acid copolymer implants on ultrasound may predict resolution of vesicoureteral reflux after injection therapy. *Clinical Radiology*, 2014; e1-e6.

[71] Higham-Kessler, J., Reinert, S. E., Snodgrass, W. T., et al. A review of failures of endoscopic treatment of vesicoureteral reflux with dextranomer microspheres. *J. Pediatr. Urol.*, Feb. 2007; 177: 710-715.

[72] Dave, S., Lorenzo, A. J., Khoury, A. E., et al. Learning from the learning curve: factors associated with successful endoscopic correction of vesicoureteral reflux using dextranomer\hyaluronic acid copolymer. *J. Urol.,* Oct. 2008; 180: 1594-1600.

[73] Routh, J. C., Reinberg, Y., Ashley, R. A., et al. Multivariate comparison of the efficacy of intraureteral versus subtrigonal techniques of dextranomer/hyaluronic acid injection. *J. Urol.*, 2007; 178: 1702- 1705.

[74] Watters, S. T., Sung, J., Skoog, S. J. Endoscopic treatment for vesicoureteral reflux: how is important is technique? *J. Pediatr. Urol.*, 2013; 9: 1192-1197.

[75] Akin, M., Erginel, B., Karadag, C. A. A comparison of the double hydrodistention implantation technique (HIT) and the HIT with a polyacrylate/polyalcohol copolymer (PPC) for the endoscopic treatment of primary vesicoureteral reflux. *Int. Urol. Nephrol.*, 2014.

[76] Capozza, N., Lais, A., Nappo, S., et al. The role of endoscopic treatment of vesicoureteral reflux: a 17-year experience. *J. Urol.*, Oct. 2004; 172: 1626-1629.

[77] Kirsch, A. J., Perez-Brayfield, M. R., Scherz, H. C. Minimally invasive treatment of vesicoureteral reflux with endoscopic injection of dextranomer/hyaluronic acid copolymer: the children's hospitals of Atlanta experience. *J. Urol.*, July 2003; 170: 211-215.

[78] Routh, J. C., Reinberg, Y. Predicting Success in the Endoscopic Management of Pediatric Vesicoureteral Reflux. *Urology*, 2010; 76: 195-198.

[79] Elder, J. S., Diaz, M. Vesicoureteral reflux: the role of bladder and bowel dysfunction. *Nature Reviews Urology*, Nov. 2013; 10: 640-648.

[80] Capozza, N., Lais, A., Matarazzo, E., et al. Influence of voiding dysfunction on the outcome of endoscopic treatment for vesicoureteral reflux. *J. Urol.*, Oct. 2002; 168: 1695-1698.

[81] Holmdahl, G., Brandstrom, P., Lackgren, G., et al. The Swedish reflux trial in children: II. Vesicoureteral reflux outcome. *J. Urol.*, 2010; 184: 280-5.

[82] Chertin, B., Arafeh, W. A., Kocherov, S. Endoscopic correction of complex cases of vesicoureteral reflux utilizing Vantris as a new non-biodegradable tissue-augmenting substance. *Pediatr. Surg. Int.*, 2014; 30: 445-448.

[83] Bartoli, F., Niglio, F., Pastore, V., et al. Polydimethylsiloxane (macroplastique®) injection for vesicoureteral reflux in duplex ureters: a comparison with single renal systems. *J. Pediatr. Urol.*, Oct. 2011; 7(5): 516-519.

[84] Akiki, A., Boissier, R., Delaport, V., et al. Endoscopic treatment of symptomatic vesicoureteral reflux after renal transplantation. *J. Urol.*, 2014, in press.

[85] Ranchin, B., Chapuis, F., Dawhara, M., et al. Vesicoureteral reflux after kidney transplantation in children. *Nephrol. Dial. Transplant.*, Nov. 2000; 15(11): 1852-8.

[86] Heckler, A. M., Sung, J., Watters, S., et al. The long-term incidence of urinary tract infection after endoscopic management of vesicoureteral reflux. *Urology*, 2014; 83(6): 1383-1387.

[87] Chi, A., Gupta, A., Snodgrass, W. Urinary tract infection following successful dextranomer/hyaluronic acid injection for vesicoureteral reflux. *J. Urol.*, 2008; 179: 1966-1969.

[88] Kandem, A. F., Giacomo, G., Aubert, D. Long-term incidence of febrile UTI after DxHA treatment of VUR. *J. Pediatr. Urol.*, 2014; 10: 56-61.

[89] Alizadeh, F., Mazdak, H., Korrami, M. H., et al. Postoperative ureteral obstruction after endoscopic treament of vesicoureteral reflux with polyacrylate polyalcohol copolymer (Vantris). *J. Pediatr. Urol.*, 2013; 9: 488-492.

[90] Al-Hunayan, A. A., Kehinde, E. O., Elsalam, M. A., Al-Mukhtar, R. S. Outcome of endoscopic treatment for vesicoureteral reflux in children using polydimethylsiloxane. *J. Urol.*, Nov. 2002; 168(5): 2181-2183.

[91] Garcia-Aparicio, L., Rodo, J., Palazon, P., et al. Acute and delayed vesicoureteral obstruction after endoscopic treatment of primary vesicoureteral reflux with dextranomer\hyaluronic acid copolymer: why and how to manage. *J. Pediatr. Urol.*, 2013; 9: 493-497.

[92] Vandersteen, D. R., Routh, J. C., Kirsch, A. J., et al. Postoperative ureteral obstruction after sub- ureteral injection of dextranomer/ hyaluronic acid copolymer. *J. Urol.*, 2006; 176: 1593.

[93] Kempf, C., Winkelmann, B., Roigas, J., et al. Severe complications after endoscopic injection of polydimethylsiloxane for the treatment of vesicoureteral reflux in early childhood. *Scand. J. Urol. Nephrol.*, 2010; 44: 347.

[94] Lorenzo, A. J., Khoury, A. E. Endoscopic treatment of reflux: management pros and cons. *Current opinion in Urology*, July 2006; 16: 299-304.

[95] Gargollo, P. C., Paltiel, H. J., Rosoklija, I., et al. Mound calcification after endoscopic treatment of vesicoureteral reflux with autologous chondrocytes-A normal variant of mound appearance? *J. Urol.*, June 2009; 181: 2702-2708.

[96] Nepple, K. G., Knudson, M. J., Cooper, C. S., et al. Symptomatic calcification of subureteral collagen ten yers after injection, *Urology*, 2007; 69(5): 982.

[97] Smith, D. P., Beegle, B. E., Noe, H. N., et al. Does technique or material used affect bladder tissue reactions when injecting Teflon or silicone paste? *Urology*, 1996; 48: 119.

[98] Palagiri, A. V. and Dangle, P. P. Distal ureteral calcification secondary to Deflux injection: a reality or myth? *Urology* 2011; 77: 1217.

[99] Nelson, C. P., Chow, J. S. Dextranomer/hyaluronic acid copolymer (Deflux) implants mimicking distal ureteral calculi on CT. *Pediatr. Radiol.*, 2008; 38: 104-106.

[100] Yankovic, F., Swartz, R., Cuckow, P., et al. Incidence of Deflux calcification masquerading as distal ureteric calculi on ultrasound. *J. Pediatr. Urol.,* 2013; 9: 820-824.

In: Vesicoureteral Reflux and Pyelonephritis
Editor: Leanna P. Newport
ISBN: 978-1-63463-497-7

Chapter IV

Up-Regulation of Tissue and Urinary Uroplakin mRNAs in Congenital Vesicoureteral Reflux

Tatsuhiro Yoshiki[1,2], Hideaki Iwaki[2], Ken-ichi Kobayashi[2], Susumu Kageyama[2], Hiromi Ii[1] and Akihiro Kawauchi[2]

[1]Department of Clinical Oncology, Kyoto Pharmaceutical University
[2]Department of Urology, Shiga University of Medical Science

Abstract

Aim: Uroplakins (UPs) are urothelium-specific transmembrane proteins consisting of the following four families: uroplakin Ia (UPIa), uroplakin Ib (UPIb), uroplakin II (UPII), and uroplakin III (UPIII). Vesicoureteral reflux (VUR) is the most common congenital urinary tract anomaly. This disease can pose a major threat to the kidneys as twenty percent of patients with endstage renal disease are reported to have VUR. Although genetic studies for *uroplakins* (*UPs*) using mouse have been reported recently, no study has focused on *UP* genes expression in VUR patients. We describe here the up-regulation of *UPs* mRNA in exfoliated urinary cells from primary VUR patients.

Methods: A real-time RT-PCR for *UPs* mRNA was performed on exfoliated urothelial cells from primary VUR and control samples. *UPs* mRNA copies were calculated for each sample. The statistical differences were assessed by the Mann-Whitney U test. Receiver operator characteristic curves were constructed for analysis of the diagnostic values.

Results: In the tissues, *UPs* gene expressions were significantly up-regulated in VUR samples relative to controls. Considering our results, all of the UP gene expressions were up-regulated in the VUR tissues. Moreover, *UPs* mRNA was found to be up-regulated to a greater extent in VUR than in control exfoliated urinary cells. In evaluating the measurement of urinary *UPs* mRNA as a screening test for VUR, the sensitivity and the specificity could be determined by the best diagnostic cutoff point.

Discussion : Regarding *UPs* mRNA in VUR, two studies of *UPII* and *UPIII* gene knockout mouse models were reported. All of the unaffected *UP* transcripts were shown by Northern blotting to be up-regulated. Though these studies were in mice, the findings are compatible with our results in humans. Our studies may have less impact because the control subjects were not age-matched. However, we submit that UPs and our results can lead to clarifying the etiology of VUR in the future. Further studies are needed of samples obtained from age- adjusted pediatric patients with other urological conditions, such as cystitis, pyelonephritis, and congenital hydronephrosis. We also investigated by a (99m) technetium dimercaptosuccinic acid renal scan the relationship between *UP* mRNA expression and the degree of renal scarring in VUR tissue samples. Although not significant, higher expression levels were found for *UP* mRNAs with the increasing degree of renal scarring.

These results show the feasibility of quantitative measurements for urinary *UP* mRNAs and the potential use in screening for VUR. In addition, our preliminary studies of RT-PCR for tissue *UP* mRNAs can be useful in elucidating the underlying mechanisms leading to VUR in the future.

Conclusions: We submit that the quantitative measurement of urinary *Ups* mRNA has a potential of developing into the first non-invasive screening test for VUR.

Keywords: Uroplakins, PCR, gene expression, up-regulation, vesicoureteral reflux

Introduction

Vesicoureteral reflux (VUR) is the most common congenital urinary anomaly in children with a reported prevalence of approximately 1% on the basis of investigations in children with a urinary tract infection (UTI) [1]. However, overall incidence of latent VUR in the Caucasian population is probably best estimated at greater than 10% according to a review of the literature [2] [3]. VUR may pose a major threat to the kidneys, which is referred to as reflux nephropathy, that can account for as much as 20% of cases with end-stage renal failure [4].

Uroplakins (UPs) are urothelium-specific transmembrane proteins, that are present in the apical surface membrane of umbrella cells [5] [6] [7]. To date, four UPs, uroplakin Ia (UPIa), uroplakin Ib (UPIb), uroplakin II (UPII), and uroplakin III (UPIII), have been found. They are packed hexagonally and form urothelial plaques that cover almost the entire apical surface of the superficial urothelium.

Although the detailed physiological roles of UPs are not clear, they are considered to stabilize the urothelial surface or to have a permeability barrier function in the urothelial membrane.

VUR has reportedly been demonstrated in a mouse knockout model of the *UPIII* gene [8], although candidate genes for the etiology of VUR have not been elucidated. However, in recent studies, no pathogenic *UPIII* mutations were identified in patients with primary VUR, including those with a family history [9, 10]. In these reports, it is seriously critical that *UPIII* mRNA was never examined, though only genetic mutations were shown.

On the basis of these findings, focusing on the changes in *UPIII* gene regulation in primary VUR patients, we recently showed a high level of *UPIII* mRNA expression in VUR urothelial tissues using a real-time reverse transcription-polymerase chain reaction (RT-PCR) approach. Furthermore, we suggested that the quantitative measurement of *UPIII* mRNA levels in urine can be developed into a non-invasive screening test for VUR [11]. In our previous report, we presented preliminary data indicating that the tissue mRNA expression of the remaining UPs was up-regulated in VUR patients. Regarding the expression of UPs mRNA in VUR, two studies have reported the expression of the *UPII* [12] and *UPIII* genes [8] in mouse knockout models. In these reports, the other unaffected UPs were shown to be expressed at high levels by Northern blotting. However, no studies describing the quantitative analysis of UPs gene expression have been reported in VUR patients, other than the expression of *UPIII* that we described previously [11].

In this study, we demonstrate the up-regulation of *UPIa*, *UPIb*, *UPII* and *UPIII* mRNA in VUR tissues using real-time RT-PCR. In addition, we show that, similar to *UPIII* [11], *UP1b* mRNA can be measured quantitatively in urinary exfoliated cells from VUR patients.

Methods

Tissue and Urine Samples

In the present study, we assessed the same tissue and urine samples that we used in the previous examination [11]. For the tissue samples, primary VUR urothelium samples greater than grade III and control bladder urothelium samples were collected from adult patients, including those with benign prostatic hyperplasia, prostate cancer, or solitary bladder tumor. The VUR samples were from adult and pediatric patients. All of these tissue samples were obtained surgically. After the tissue samples were excised during the course of surgery, they were stored immediately at -80°C until use. These urine samples were obtained from patients who had visited the urological outpatients department or healthy volunteers. Three urine samples that were contaminated with leukocytes at 5–10 cells/high power field were included. The urine samples were centrifuged for 10 min at 1,500 rpm to collect exfoliated cells and washed with phosphate-buffered saline. The urinary cell pellets were stored immediately at -80°C until use. The diagnosis of VUR had been confirmed by voiding cystography and the detection of renal scarring in VUR patients had been assessed by a (99m) technetium dimercaptosuccinic acid (DMSA) renal scan.

Informed consent was obtained from all patients and the study was conducted in accordance with the requirements of our Institutional Research and Human Rights Committee.

cDNA Preparation

cDNA synthesis was performed as described previously [11]. Briefly, total RNA was extracted using TRIzol Reagent (Invitrogen, Carlsbad, CA, USA) and RNA was reverse transcribed by SuperscriptII (Invitrogen, Carlsbad, CA, USA) using random primers (Takara Biomedical, Otsu, Japan) according to the manufacturer's instructions. The integrity of the synthesized cDNA was confirmed by amplification of the housekeeping gene glyceraldehyde-3-phosphate dehydrogenase (*GAPDH*). The prepared cDNA samples were stored at -20°C until used for RT-PCR.

Real-Time RT-PCR for *UPIa, UPIb*, *UPII* and *UPIII* mRNA

Quantitative measurements of tissue and urinary UPs were performed as described previously [11]. Briefly, real-time RT-PCR was performed on the LightCycler™ system (Roche Diagnostics, Indianapolis, IN, USA) using LightCycler FastStart DNA Master SYBR GREEN I according to the manufacturer's instructions. The PCR profiles and primers are published previously [11,14]. After amplification, melting curves were obtained by holding the temperature at 7°C higher than the respective annealing temperature. Serial 10-fold dilutions of gel purified PCR products were used for the standard DNA and they were included in each run. The concentrations of the transcripts per reaction mixture were measured using LightCycler™ software with reference to the standard DNA. The values for each UP transcripts were then normalized to that of GAPDH and the mRNA copies were calculated for each sample. All tests were performed in duplicate to ensure reproducibility.

Data Analysis

Data analysis was performed with SPSS II for Windows software (SPSS Japan Inc., Tokyo, Japan). Statistical difference was assessed by the Mann-Whitney U test. Significance was defined as $p < 0.05$.

Results

Quantitative PCR for *UPIa, UPIb*, *UPII* and *UPIII* mRNA in Tissue

UPIa, UPIb, *UPII* and *UPIII* gene expression was examined in urothelial tissues from primary VUR and control subjects (Table 1) using real-time quantitative PCR analysis. The levels of all UP mRNA were significantly higher in the VUR tissue samples than in the controls. The mean ± SE values for the VUR and control samples were 11513.5 ± 4491.3 vs. 677.8 ± 360.4 for *UPIa* ($p < 0.001$), 9634.1 ± 3653.4 vs. 841.7 ± 356.7 for *UPIb* ($p = 0.001$), 1700.0 ± 528.7 vs. 131.9 ± 70.0 for *UPII* ($p = 0.001$), respectively.

Table 1. Comparison of quantified relative values of tissue or urine *uroplakin(UP)* mRNA expression

		UP Ia			*UP Ib*			*UP II*		
		(mRNA copies)			(mRNA copies)			(mRNA copies)		
Sample	n	Mean ±SE	Median	P value	Mean ±SE	Median	P value	Mean ±SE	Median	P value
VUR (tissue)	20	11513.5 ±4491.3	2716.7	<0.001	9634.1 ±3653.4	2752.3	0.001	1700.0 ±528.7	642.85	0.001
Control (tissue)	11	677.8 ±360.4	96.4		841.7 ±356.7	213.3		131.9 ±70.0	37.1	
VUR (tissue): No. of scarring										
None	8	30162.5 ±27326.7	2958.1		21260.5 ±18821.7	2752.3		5070.3 ±4474.0	642.9	
One site	4	4647.0 ±1675.0	4369.0		4169.6 ±1589.6	3070.7		1396.2 ±575.3	1289.1	
Two or more	7	19315.9 ±10144.3	10960.1		14117.4 ±6583.7	6594.4		2122.7 ±845.9	1501.5	
VUR (urine)	18				989.4 ±396.4	430.8	0.017			
Control (urine)	20				264.1 ±66.0	125.9				

* P<0.05 is statistically significant as assessed by Mann-Whitney U test. SE: standard error.

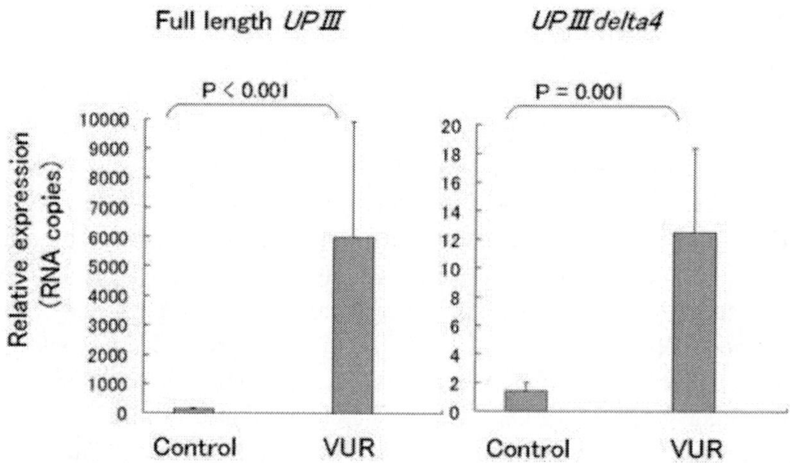

Figure 1. Quantification of urinary *UPIII* mRNA expression in vesicoureteral reflux (VUR) ($n = 21$) and control patients ($n = 38$). *UPIIIdelta4* means a novel alternative splicing variant of *UPIII* which lost the exon 4.

The median values were 28-fold higher for *UPIa* (2716.7 vs. 96.4), 13-fold higher for *UPIb* (2752.3 vs. 213.3) and 17-fold higher for *UPII* (642.9 vs. 37.1) than in the control samples. Even when 3 age-matched adult VUR patients and 11 controls were compared, significantly higher expression levels of *UPIa, UPIb*, and *UPII* were also seen in the VUR patients. These results showed that the expression of all of the other UP genes, in addition to *UPIII*, was up-regulated to a greater extent in the VUR tissue samples than in the controls (Figure 1).

Relationship between UP mRNA Expression and Renal Scarring in VUR Patients

We also evaluated the relationship between UP mRNA expression and the degree of renal scarring in VUR tissue samples. Among the 20 VUR patients, 19 cases were assessed for renal scarring using a DMSA renal scan. There were 8 patients with no scarring, 4 patients with 1 site of scarring, and 7 patients with 2 or more sites of scarring. In this order, the median values of UP mRNA copies were 2958.1, 4369.0, and 10960.1 for *UPIa*, 2752.3, 3070.7, and 6594.4 for *UPIb*, and 642.9, 1289.1, and 1501.5 for *UPII*. Although a significant difference was not seen, higher expression levels were found for *UPIa, UPIb*, and *UPII* mRNA with the increasing degree of renal scarring.

Quantitative Measurement of Urinary *UPIb* and *UPIII* mRNA Levels

Following on from our previous study of urinary *UPIII* mRNA levels [11], we performed real-time quantitative PCR analysis of *UPIb* mRNA using exfoliated urinary cells from 18 VUR patients and 20 controls. *UPIb* transcripts were detected in all VUR and control samples. Significantly higher levels of *UPIb* mRNA or *UPIII* were detected in urine samples from VUR patients than in the control urine samples (mean ± SE: 989.4 ± 396.4 vs. 264.1 ± 66.0 for *UPIb* ($p = 0.017$), 438.5±180.0 vs. 70.8±12.8 for *UPIII* ($p = 0.004$), respectively, Figure 1). *UPIb* transcripts ranged from 67.1 to 6058.5 copies with a median value of 430.8 in the VUR patients, and from 12.1 to 1133.6 copies with a median value of 125.9 in the control patients. These results verify the feasibility of the quantitative measurement of mRNA in urine and support the probability of establishing a urine test for VUR that we described previously [11].

Discussion

Both our studies demonstrated the up-regulation of *UPIa, UPIb*, *UPII* and *UPIII* mRNA in urothelial tissues from patients with VUR compared to those from controls.

In the report of a *UPIII* gene knockout mouse [8], *UPIa, UPIb*, and *UPII* transcripts, which were the unaffected genes, were shown to be up-regulated by Northern blotting. Similarly, the expression of *UPIa, UPIb*, and *UPIII* mRNA was enhanced in another study of a *UPII* gene knockout mouse [12]. Considering these findings from the knockout mouse models, our findings of the overexpression of all of the UPs in VUR tissue might be expected. However, our studies are meaningful in that the up-regulation of UP mRNA in VUR tissue was demonstrated in terms of quantitative measurements.

Our study showed that increased levels of *UPIa, UPIb*, and *UPII* mRNA were associated with the degree of renal scarring. In this regard, we had mentioned a similar finding for *UPIII* mRNA expression in our previous report (data not shown) [11]. Recently, the utility of a top-down approach, which focuses on identifying reflux-related renal scarring before more invasive imaging is considered, has been discussed for children with a UTI, including VUR patients [13]. Renal scarring is a significant sign for high grade

(III or greater) VUR. If a non-invasive urine test can be used to predict renal scarring, it will be a valuable clinical tool because VUR patients with renal scarring could be identified and treated. Although further study on a larger population is needed, our results suggest that the measurement of UP mRNA expression may develop into a useful marker for renal scarring in VUR patients.

We previously suggested the usefulness of measuring urinary *UPIII* mRNA levels as a screening test for VUR. In addition, we have now shown that the up-regulation of urinary *UPIb* mRNA levels was detectable using exfoliated urinary cells, similar to *UPIII*. Thus, our study verified that quantitative RT-PCR using urinary exfoliated cells is feasible in the clinical setting. In the etiology of VUR, it seems to be undoubtedly that the dysregulation of UP expression plays an important role. The results of previous reports of mouse knockout models of *UPIII* [8] and *UPII* [12] suggest a correlation between a deficiency of UPs and the development of VUR. However, we demonstrated the up-regulation of UP mRNA expression in human VUR tissues using quantitative real-time RT-PCR. The discrepancy between these gene ablation and mRNA overexpression studies may suggest that there are unknown molecules with negative feedback regulation against the production of UPs. Considering the overexpression of all four UPs, it is possible that a common regulatory mechanism may control the transcription of UPs. Our results are considered to be meaningful to elucidate the mechanism of VUR, which may lead to the development of an effective treatment for this condition. In conclusion, we demonstrated the up-regulation of mRNA for all four UPs in VUR tissues using real-time RT-PCR in our previous [11] and present reports. In addition, we have shown that quantitative RT-PCR using urinary exfoliated cells is feasible for the analysis of *UPIb* mRNA levels, following on from our previous study on the expression of *UPIII* mRNA [11]. Although further studies are needed, we believe that our data have significance to elucidate the underlying mechanism of VUR and to establish a valuable screening test for VUR.

References

[1] Bailey R. Vesicoureteric reflux in healthy infants and children. In: Hodson J, Kincaid-Smith P (eds) Reflux nephropathy. Masson, New York, 1979; 59-61.

[2] Atala A, Keating MA. Vesicoureteral reflux and megaureter. In: Walsh PC, Retik AB, Vaughan D, Vein AJ (eds) Campbell's Urology (8th ed). WB Saunders, Philadelphia, 2002; 2053-116.

[3] Sargent MA. What is the normal prevalence of vesicoureteral reflux? *Pediatr. Radiol.* 2000; 30: 587-93.

[4] Gordon I. Vesico-ureteric reflux, urinary-tract infection, and renal damage in children. *Lancet* 1995; 346: 489-90.

[5] Yu J, Manabe M, Wu XR, Xu C, Surya B, Sun TT. Uroplakin I: a 27-kD protein associated with the asymmetric unit membrane of mammalian urothelium. *J. Cell Biol.* 1990; 111: 1207-16.

[6] Wu XR, Manabe M, Yu J, Sun TT. Large scale purification and immunolocalization of bovine uroplakins I, II, and III. Molecular markers of urothelial differentiation. *J. Biol. Chem.* 1990; 265: 19170-9.

[7] Wu XR, Medina JJ, Sun TT. Selective interactions of UPIa and UPIb, two members of the transmembrane 4 superfamily, with distinct single transmembrane-domained proteins in differentiated urothelial cells. *J. Biol. Chem.* 1995; 270: 29752-9.

[8] Hu P, Deng FM, Liang FX, Hu CM, Auerbach AB, Shapiro E, Wu XR, Kachar B, Sun TT. Ablation of uroplakin III gene results in small urothelial plaques, urothelial leakage, and vesicoureteral reflux. *J. Cell Biol.* 2000; 151: 961-72.

[9] Giltay JC, van de Meerakker J, van Amstel HK, de Jong TP. No pathogenic mutations in the uroplakin III gene of 25 patients with primary vesicoureteral reflux. *J. Urol.* 2004; 171: 931-2.

[10] Jiang S, Gitlin J, Deng FM, Liang FX, Lee A, Atala A, Bauer SB, Ehrlich GD, Feather SA, Goldberg JD, Goodship JA, Goodship TH, Hermanns M, Hu FZ, Jones KE, Malcolm S, Mendelsohn C, Preston RA, Retik AB, Schneck FX, Wright V, Ye XY, Woolf AS, Wu XR, Ostrer H, Shapiro E, Yu J, Sun TT. Lack of major involvement of human uroplakin genes in vesicoureteral reflux: implications for disease heterogeneity. *Kidney Int.* 2004; 66: 10-9.

[11] Iwaki H, Johnin K, Kageyama S, Kim CJ, Isono T, Yoshiki T. Up-regulation of urinary UPIII mRNA levels in vesicoureteral reflux patients: potential application as a screening test for vesicoureteral reflux. *Int. J. Urol.* 2007;14:918-23.

[12] Kong XT, Deng FM, Hu P, Liang FX, Zhou G, Auerbach AB, Genieser N, Nelson PK, Robbins ES, Shapiro E, Kachar B, Sun TT. Roles of uroplakins in plaque formation, umbrella cell enlargement, and urinary tract diseases. *J. Cell Biol.* 2004;167:1195-204.

[13] Pohl HG, Belman AB. The "Top-Down" Approach to the Evaluation of Children with Febrile Urinary Tract Infection. *Adv. Urol.* 2009: 783409.

[14] Iwaki H, Kageyama S, Yoshiki T. Upregulation of tissue and urinary uroplakin mRNA in patients with vesicoureteral reflux. *Int. J. Urol.* 2014 :21:347.

Index

M

N

O

P

R